Prevention's
DIABETES
BREAKTHROUGHS
2008

WALKING FIT

Prevention's
DIABETES
BREAKTHROUGHS
2008

WALKING FIT

from the editors of **Prevention** magazine

RODALE

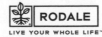

We inspire and enable people to improve their lives and the world around them

For more of our products visit **rodalestore.com** or call 800-848-4735

Contents

Part I

On the Road to Better Health

Part II

Are You Ready to Walk?

Part III
Walk in Any Weather

Part IV
Walk Off Your Weight

Part V
Strength Training for Walkers

Part VI
The Spirit in Walking

Part VII
Getting Started with Dynamic Walking

Part VIII
Everything Else You Need to Know

Introduction

Walk Away from Diabetes

Almost 75 million Americans, one in four of us, have diabetes or prediabetes. And if we continue on our present path, the diabetes epidemic will keep on gathering steam like a freight train careening downhill. Experts speculate that if present trends continue, one in three Americans born in 2000—one in two of them minorities—will develop diabetes in their lifetimes.

Clearly our present path is perilous. We need to find a new path; what we need is a walking path.

"Walking is medicine," says Michael See, MS, registered clinical exercise physiologist at the Joslin Diabetes Center in Boston. "Almost anybody can walk; it's the most popular form of exercise in our society. Yet less than half (49 percent) of Americans achieve the recommended amount of physical activity, and almost a quarter (24 percent) report no physical activity."

Exercise is important for everyone, but studies show its power to help prevent and manage diabetes. "People who walk more have less risk of diabetes, regardless of their weight," says See.

Walking is so beneficial that health organizations such as the American Diabetes Association (ADA) recommend it for disease prevention and treatment. The ADA says to aim for 30 minutes a day, at least 5 days a week, of aerobic exercise, such as brisk walking.

"The key is, walking has to be purposeful," says See. "That means it's in addition to your normal daily activities. Running after the kids, shopping at the mall, and working in a hectic office don't cut it. Even subtle ways of increasing your activity, such as taking the stairs instead of the elevator and parking farther from store entrances to walk farther, aren't replacements for purposeful exercise."

Stephen G. Rosen, MD, chief of endocrinology at Pennsylvania Hospital in Philadelphia, says, "With a regular walking program, some people may be able to come off of their diabetes medicine entirely."

Ready to lace up your walking shoes and get going? This book is the definitive guide to walking with diabetes, offering the tools and techniques to help you walk farther and faster, with greater comfort and less risk of injury.

Part I offers strong motivation to step off into your walking program. You'll learn how walking can help you fight diabetes, heart disease, arthritis, back problems, and even stress. Once you have the will, Part II will show you the way. You'll find out how to choose the best walking shoes and gear and determine the best walking place and time.

In Part III of the book, we'll eliminate some well-worn excuses for not walking. You'll learn how to beat the heat, brave the cold, and survive the sneezin' season. Part IV offers advice to help you pare down the pounds. You'll find shape-up plans, great gadgets for boosting your burn, and a walker's guide to eating for weight loss.

The perfect complement to your new walking program is a little strength training. And Part V is where you'll find it. Stand taller, sculpt sexy arms, cinch your waist, firm your legs, and more. It's simple: Move some weights to get rid of your excess weight.

In Part VI, we'll talk about some special types of walking. Get in touch with nature and yourself with sky walking, labyrinth walking, creative walking, and nature walking. Part VII features a unique type of walking: Dynamic Walking. This walking system can help anyone get more out of walking, no matter what their speed, fitness level, or health status. It's a whole new way to walk, for a whole new you. Finally in Part VIII, we'll wind it all up with answers to the most popular walking questions.

We hope this book offers you the education, inspiration, and motivation to walk away from diabetes. Ready, set, go! Let's take that first step on your new walking path.

ON THE ROAD
TO BETTER HEALTH

CHAPTER 1

WALKING IS POWERFUL MEDICINE

Whether you're just starting a walking program or you're already a regular walker, your health likely played a role in your decision to get fit. Maybe you've recently been diagnosed with diabetes or you're concerned because your blood sugar control isn't what it should be. Perhaps you want to lose a few pounds or protect your heart from disease or keep your bones strong and your joints limber. Walking can do all this and more.

But when we talk about walking for health, we must look beyond the physical benefits. After all, health is a rich fabric spun from physical, mental, emotional, and spiritual threads. If one of these threads becomes frayed for any reason, it can weaken the entire fabric. What you eat, how much you sleep, how you handle your personal and professional relationships, how you view the world and your place in it—all of these things influence whether or not you feel vital and strong. They also have a real impact on your body.

The same can be said of walking. It supports health in every sense— physically, mentally, emotionally, and spiritually. It enriches and balances your life. And it just plain makes you feel good. No wonder the Greek physician Hippocrates (460–377 BC) deemed walking to be "man's best medicine."

FENDING OFF DIABETES

"Exercise does a lot for people with diabetes," says Kashif Munir, MD, an endo-crinologist and medical director of the Joslin Diabetes Center at Baltimore

Washington Medical Center in Glen Burnie, Maryland. "Long-term exercise improves blood glucose and blood pressure and reduces the risk of heart disease. It also relieves stress and tension, and it improves muscle tone, strength, and flexibility.

"For most people, walking will improve your blood sugar levels right away and for the next several hours," Dr. Munir continues. "In fact, studies have shown that exercise can improve insulin sensitivity for up to 48 hours."

That's important because diabetes is a disease of high levels of blood sugar resulting from defects of insulin production, insulin action, or both. It can lead to serious complications, including death. But fortunately people with diabetes can take steps to control their disease and to lower their risk of its complications, such as cardiovascular disease; walking is one-step shopping for both.

"Walking is one of the simplest and safest means of treating diabetes and promoting cardiovascular health," says Janet Bond Brill, PhD, RD, LDN, a nutritionist, exercise physiologist, and National Strength and Conditioning Association certified personal trainer in Miami. According to Dr. Brill, here are some of the benefits associated with a regular program of aerobic exercise, such as walking, for people with diabetes.

- Lowers LDL or "bad" cholesterol
- Raises HDL or "good" cholesterol
- Targets abdominal or visceral "belly fat"
- Promotes production of disease-fighting antioxidants within vessel walls
- Cuts risk of stroke
- Helps with weight loss and maintenance of weight loss
- Increases cells' ability to utilize insulin

We'll talk more about the why, when, and where of walking with diabetes in later chapters. But for now, know that the American Diabetes Association (ADA) recommends that people with diabetes aim for 30 minutes of exercise a day, such as a brisk walk, at least 5 days a week. If you haven't been very active, the ADA suggests starting out with 5 to 10 minutes a day and adding some more time each week or splitting up your activity throughout the day.

BOOSTING IMMUNITY, ONE STEP AT A TIME

To get a complete picture of how walking supports good health, you must start at the cellular level. A daily walk keeps certain cells—your immune cells—tuned up for action, ready to whip viruses and battle bacteria. In fact, some experts believe that walking may be one of your best weapons for fighting off infection and disease and getting on the road to recovery fast.

Strong statement? Maybe. But a number of studies have shown that a moderate walk not only relieves the stress that may trigger or aggravate an illness but also stimulates your immune system, your body's main defense against disease. In one such study, a 45-minute walk (about 3 miles) increased the activity of certain immune cells by about 57 percent. The cells' activity level returned to normal about 3 hours after the walk.

Now researchers don't know for sure whether walking can make you heal faster, but some studies suggest that people who walk consistently (meaning, every day) develop fewer illnesses than people who are sedentary. The fact that walking is a moderate activity may be key to its immunity-enhancing effects. Indeed, other studies show that long bouts of intense exercise—such as an hour of pavement-pounding, heavy-breathing running—can actu-

ally suppress your immune system and make you more susceptible to infection.

This brings up a common question walkers have: When you're under the weather, should you continue your walking program or take off a few days until you feel better? One expert recommends this rule of thumb: If you have a headache or runny nose, or if you're sneezing, you're okay to walk as long as your temperature is normal. In cases of fever, sore throat, or coughing, you should rest until your symptoms subside.

Even if you feel well enough to continue walking, skip the marathons, races, and fun walks for the time being—unless you have your doctor's okay to participate.

GAINING GROUND AGAINST CANCER

If walking has a beneficial effect on the immune system, then might it have some protective effect against any type of cancer? The research so far seems promising.

In one study, laboratory rats were given a chemical that induces breast cancer. Half of the rats were put in cages that allowed them free access to an exercise wheel. The rats could run on the wheel any time they got the urge, and they did so frequently. These rats developed one-third fewer cases of breast cancer than the rats that didn't have a wheel. What's more, their tumors appeared much later.

Exercise in general keeps cropping up as a factor in cancer prevention and treatment. Scientists don't yet understand how exercise might deter tumors, but they do know that people who work out regularly seem to get cancer less often than those who don't.

For instance, three separate population studies found that men with physically demanding jobs—such as carpenters, plumbers, gardeners, and mail carriers—are less prone to colon cancer than men who sit all day. In another study, Harvard University researchers determined that men who engage in about an hour of vigorous activity every day reduce their risk of prostate cancer by 47 to 88 percent. And researchers at the University of Iowa Cancer Center in Iowa City found that women over age 65, a group that accounts for 50 percent of all breast cancer cases, are less likely to get the disease if they exercise moderately. In fact, the more active these women are, the lower their chances of being diagnosed with breast cancer are.

While no one can say for certain that walking every day protects against all kinds of cancer, enough evidence has been uncovered to persuade the American Cancer Society to recommend regular exercise as one possible way to reduce your risk. And if you or someone you know is receiving treatment for cancer, walking may be the ticket to a steady recovery and the speedy return of strength and energy.

For example, walking may counteract the fatigue and weakness that are associated with high-dose chemotherapy. Traditionally, patients have been told to rest to recuperate from chemo. But extended bed rest leads to loss of muscle strength and cardiovascular fitness, which only worsens fatigue and weakness—so much so that these problems can linger for years after treatment. So a team of German researchers tried a different approach: They encouraged patients to exercise regularly after completing chemotherapy. People had not only more energy but also a more positive attitude toward recovery.

The benefits of exercise for cancer patients are psychological as well as physical. One study of women being treated for breast cancer showed that their levels of depression and anxiety dropped dramatically after 10 weeks of regular exercise—30 to 40 minutes, 4 days a week. This finding is especially encouraging because breast cancer survivors face a significant risk of depression and anxiety.

WHAT ELSE CAN WALKING DO FOR YOU?

To be sure, scientists have only begun to scratch the surface in understanding the benefits of exercise—not only for battling diabetes, boosting immunity, and fighting cancer, but also for enhancing all aspects of health. Interestingly, most studies of exercise use walking as the activity of choice. And they have revealed some extraordinary information about what this most fundamental of workouts can do.

- It supports weight loss and weight maintenance.
- It reduces the risk of heart disease and stroke.
- It eases the pain and stiffness of arthritis.
- It keeps bones strong, which prevents osteoporosis.
- In women, it relieves premenstrual and menopausal discomforts.
- It improves sleep.
- It builds strength, flexibility, and stamina.
- It enhances mental function.
- It counteracts anger, depression, and anxiety.

We'll take a closer look at some of these benefits in the chapters that follow. But as you can see, you have a lot to gain just from lacing up a pair of walking shoes and putting one foot in front of the other.

CHAPTER 2

THE BEST DEFENSE AGAINST DIABETES

For some reason, the word *diabetes* doesn't strike fear in the hearts of most Americans. But it should. According to the American Diabetes Association, about 7 percent of Americans, 20.8 million of us, have diabetes. Unfortunately, 6.2 million people (or nearly one-third) are unaware that they have the disease. Even more staggering, 54 million people have prediabetes, which is blood glucose levels higher than normal but not high enough to be classified as diabetes; it's a condition that raises the risk of developing type 2 diabetes.

Not surprisingly, given these statistics, diabetes is the fifth-leading cause of death in the United States. In fact, since 1987, the death rate due to diabetes has increased by 45 percent, while the death rates due to heart disease, stroke, and cancer have all declined.

Even worse, experts think that these figures for diabetes are too low. Studies show that diabetes is generally underreported on death certificates, especially for older folks who had multiple chronic conditions. Because of this, the death toll from diabetes is believed to be much higher than officially reported.

One of the terrible ironies of diabetes is that by the time you find out you have it, it has been wreaking havoc in your body for several years, gumming up blood vessels, damaging organs, and starving your body

Danger Signs

Most people don't give much thought to their feet, until there's a problem. People with diabetes, however, don't have that luxury.

"The longer a person has diabetes, the more likely certain complications of their feet can develop," says John M. Giurini, DPM, president-elect of the American College of Foot and Ankle Surgeons and associate professor in surgery at Harvard Medical School in Boston. "The first complication is loss of sensation. People with diabetes and absent sensation can develop blisters, cuts and sores, and stress fractures and not feel them. So these problems can go untreated.

"The second complication that can develop, especially with long-term diabetes, is problems with circulation," he continues. "People have diminished bloodflow to their feet. Then if they develop a problem, such as a blister or sore, it may not heal as easily."

Check your feet often for the following possible signs and symptoms, says Robert Katz, DPM, a podiatrist in Bradenton, Florida.

- Numbness
- Redness
- Tingling sensations
- Burning sensations
- Loss of hair on the toes
- Cuts and scrapes that are slow to heal

Also watch out for bruising that could indicate an injury, unexplained swelling, clear or bloody drainage, and pain, if you have normal sensation, adds Dr. Giurini. "These are all signs that something may be going on that needs attention."

of energy. Left untreated, diabetes can set the stage for a host of health problems, including heart attack, stroke, kidney disease, blindness, impotence, and limb amputation.

Do we have your attention? Good! Because there's one more fact that you need to know: Even if you already have diabetes, you can control the disease and avoid many of its consequences. "If you come close to doing the right thing, there's no reason you shouldn't live out a normal life," says Gerald Bernstein, MD, associate clinical professor of medicine at Albert Einstein College of Medicine of Yeshiva University in Bronx, New York. "To me, normal means age 90."

And what's the "right thing" that Dr. Bernstein alludes to? You can probably guess: Eat better and *exercise*.

THE EXERCISE–INSULIN CONNECTION

"Walking helps people with diabetes in several ways," says Stephen G. Rosen, MD, chief of endocrinology at Pennsylvania Hospital in Philadelphia. "It makes the body more sensitive to insulin, and therefore it improves blood glu-cose control, and it also helps with weight loss. As your weight comes down, your body uses insulin more effectively, so you may not need as much medicine for your diabetes."

To what does exercise owe its protective effects? First, it actually increases the number of insulin receptors on your cells. Insulin helps blood sugar move into cells, where it needs to go. Otherwise, it just sloshes around in your bloodstream, gumming up the blood vessel walls like a little kid who has dunked his hands in a jar of honey.

If you've already been diagnosed with diabetes, regular exercise can help control the progression of the disease. People who take insulin may be able to reduce the amount of medication they need, as physical activity enables their bodies to use insulin more efficiently.

Second, exercise helps you lose some unneeded pounds. Helping you slim down is an important benefit because overweight is a major risk factor for diabetes. (By medical standards, you're considered overweight if you exceed your ideal weight by more than 20 percent.) Being overweight puts more pressure on the body's ability to use insulin to control blood sugar. Therefore, it makes it more likely for you to develop diabetes. Almost 90 percent of people with type 2 diabetes are overweight.

Studies are just starting to show the preventive power of fitness. The Nurses' Health Study, for example, found that women who worked up a sweat more than once a week reduced their risk of developing diabetes by 30 percent. And Chinese researchers determined that people with high blood sugar who engaged in moderate exercise (and made other lifestyle changes) were 40 percent less likely to develop full-blown diabetes. "It wasn't really vigorous exercise either," notes Richard Eastman, MD, former director of the diabetes division of the National Institute of Diabetes and Digestive and Kidney Diseases in Bethesda, Maryland. In other words, brisk walking would do the trick.

As a bonus, regular exercise can help keep your brain sharp. Scientists have observed that older people with diabetes sometimes have problems thinking clearly. In one study, physical activity appeared to stimulate just the type of brain activity that had become impaired. Exactly what it is about physical activity that revs up the brain hasn't been determined, and being a regular walker won't turn you into an Einstein. But some experts theorize that exercise-related brain activity could be part of the reason why some folks say they are able to solve sticky problems while they are ticking off minutes and miles on their treadmills.

For all of these reasons, exercise may be one of the best diabetes therapies around. And one of the best forms of exercise is walking.

GETTING STARTED, SAFELY

"Before people with diabetes who haven't been exercising begin a walking program, they should discuss it with their doctors," says Kashif Munir, MD, an endocrinologist and medical director of the Joslin Diabetes Center at Baltimore Washington Medical Center in Glen Burnie, Maryland. "This is especially true if they have cardiovascular risk factors, such as chest discomfort or shortness of breath. They might need a stress test or an evaluation of their heart to make sure it's safe to start an exercise program."

An important factor to discuss with your doctor before you start walking if you have diabetes is your medication.

In Step with Richard Daly

He Got Off Medicine with Exercise

When Richard Daly started his walking program in the early 1980s, he had the best of intentions. But he didn't account for the brutal winters of his native Michigan. Each year, when the temperature dropped in late fall, he'd put away his walking shoes until the following spring. His winter workouts consisted primarily of reaching for Twinkies and other treats.

"Every spring, I'd lose 18 pounds. Every winter, I'd gain about 30," Richard says. "You don't need a math degree to figure out what was happening." Unfortunately, he failed to make the calculations. Over the years, his weight climbed to 244 pounds.

That wasn't the only problem. Richard noticed that he felt tired all the time, and he had an almost unquenchable thirst. One night in April 1996, he drank eight colas in less than an hour. "The next thing I knew, I was in the hospital," he recalls. "I was diagnosed with diabetes."

Richard spent 5 days in the hospital. He learned how to give himself insulin shots to control his blood sugar. He also attended diabetes education classes, which taught him the importance of a healthy lifestyle. "Those classes inspired me to take control," he says.

On his first morning home from the hospital, Richard started a real walking

"People with diabetes need to know how their medications may affect their blood sugar," says Michael See, MS, registered clinical exercise physiologist at the Joslin Diabetes Center in Boston. "Some medications can cause low blood sugar, and since exercise makes you more sensitive to insulin, that can be a tricky combination. Ask your doctor what the appropriate range is for your blood sugar around activity."

Start your walking program slowly, says Dr. Munir. "Walk for 5 to 10 minutes a day and slowly build up to reach

program. "Every day, rain or snow, I walked for at least 35 minutes," he says. "When the weather was really bad, I walked at a local mall or on a treadmill I had bought. I also walked the 2 miles to work and home again."

Along with walking on a daily basis, Richard made some changes in his eating habits. He ditched the Twinkies and began buying whole foods such as fruits, vegetables, and whole grain breads. He also started eating oatmeal and bran cereal, with fat-free milk and raspberries or blueberries for flavor.

"I'd eat three meals a day, then snack on fruit, cottage cheese, carrots, or a bagel," Richard says. "I'd indulge once in a while, but I'd make up for it at the next meal by choosing something light and healthful."

The payoff was enormous. Within a month of his release from the hospital, Richard was off insulin and taking only a small dose of another medication. Within 2 months, he was off all drugs. He began slimming down even faster. "I actually had to add food to my diet to keep from losing too much weight," he says. "Then I started strength training three times a week."

A year after leaving the hospital, Richard was down to a lean and fit 170 pounds. His waist was 10 inches smaller. Even better, his blood sugar dropped below 100 from its highest of 290.

"My doctor still shakes his head in amazement at what I've accomplished," Richard says. "I've never felt better!"

the goal of 30 minutes a day, at least 5 days a week," he said. "Or you might evaluate your progress by counting steps instead. Wear a pedometer one week to determine how many steps you take. Then every week try to increase that, such as 3,000 steps, then 4,000, to reach a goal of 10,000 steps a day. Start low; go slow."

Start your exercise program on level ground, adds Dr. Rosen. "Don't begin by going up hills."

It's okay to build up to that 30-minutes-a-day goal slowly, especially if you've been inactive for a while. But once you're up to 30 minutes a day, you're getting into the diabetes-fighting zone. According to Dr. Bernstein, you must exercise for at least 30 minutes three times a week to enhance your body's use of insulin. If your goal is to lose weight, however, you would do well to walk five to seven times each week. (We'll talk more about weight loss later in this book.)

A word of caution: If you skip a day, don't try to make up for it by walking twice as fast or twice as far during your next workout. Vigorous exercise can actually cause blood sugar to rise, especially in people who have insulin deficiencies.

That's why it's critical that, starting the very first day you walk, you get in the habit of testing your blood sugar level before and after you walk. If you walk longer than half an hour, check it during your walk as well. Exercise affects people's blood sugar levels differently, and you need to find out how it affects yours.

When you have diabetes, the timing of your walks can help regulate your blood sugar level. On one hand, people with type 2 diabetes may benefit from exercising *before* meals, which helps control appetite and promote weight loss. On the other hand, they might want to exercise

after meals because exercise tends to lower blood sugar levels. Check with your doctor to find out what's best for you.

For people with type 1 diabetes, it's best not to exercise on an empty stomach. These folks should plan their walks for about an hour or so after a meal, when blood sugar levels are at their highest.

"People with type 1 diabetes whose blood sugar levels are high and have ketones shouldn't do any activity at that time," says Dr. Munir. "They need to get their blood sugar levels down with insulin before they exercise."

While it's true that sometimes exercise can raise your blood sugar level, other times exercise can send blood sugar plummeting. This reaction is most common among people who use insulin. Ask your doctor how much exercise you can tolerate before you need to replenish your store of carbohydrates. And carry a healthy snack—such as a piece of fresh fruit, dried fruit, or some peanuts or trail mix—with you for just this purpose.

Another thing to be sure to bring with you on your walks is plenty of water. "It's important especially for people with diabetes to stay hydrated when they exercise," says Dr. Munir. "Dehydration can increase blood sugar levels."

Put Your Feet to the Test

People with diabetes need to be extra-vigilant about foot care. A common side effect of the disease is a loss of sensation (called *diabetic neuropathy*) that can allow minor injuries to turn into major problems.

"If you can't feel a blister, you may not treat it properly," explains Linda Haas, RN, certified diabetes educator and former president of the American Diabetes Association. "The wound can become infected, which may lead to ulcerations and even amputation."

A free home test kit can help you discover if your feet are at risk for injury. Offered by the Lower Extremity Amputation Prevention (LEAP) program, the kit contains a reusable monofilament (something like a fishing line) that you press against your foot. If you can't feel the monofilament, you may be losing sensation, and you should see your doctor.

In one study, the monofilament test was accurate 87 percent of the time. To order your kit, visit www.ask.hrsa.gov/leapindividual.cfm.

In addition to using the monofilament test, you should continue to visually inspect your feet for blisters on a daily basis and especially after walking.

TAKE CARE OF THOSE TOOTSIES

Your doctor has likely told you the importance of taking care of your feet. Not only is it important, it's imperative for someone with diabetes. Any small blister or sore can turn into a life- or limb-threatening condition.

Unfortunately, people with diabetes often have difficulty feeling problems on their feet because of nerve damage associated with the condition. To complicate matters, they're also more prone to infection. Even the slightest irritation left untreated can lead to major complications. So if you're launching a walking program, you want to do what you can to keep your feet healthy.

"People with diabetes starting a

walking program should have a foot evaluation by a foot and ankle specialist to determine their level of circulation, level of sensation, and any potential foot deformities that could lead to problems," says John M. Giurini, DPM, president-elect of the American College of Foot and Ankle Surgeons and associate professor in surgery at Harvard Medical School in Boston. "Once their risk level is determined, they can be properly educated about preventive care, foot gear, and the best type of exercise for them."

Above all else, that means investing in good-fitting walking shoes and comfortable socks. (See "Shoe-Shopping Strategies" on page 58.)

As you begin your walking program, get into the habit of inspecting your feet on a daily basis. "If you have diabetes, you should do a foot exam before each and every walk," adds Dr. Rosen. (See "Danger Signs" on page 9.)

Also take a close look at your shoes before you slip your feet into them. "To prevent problems, before each walk, thoroughly inspect inside your shoes," says Dr. Giurini. "A foreign object in a shoe—such as a pebble or a tack coming through the shoe—could cause trauma to the foot that will need to be looked at by a doctor."

Be mindful of the condition of your feet and shoes as you walk. Keep your feet dry to discourage the formation of blisters and never walk in wet shoes. If you notice any irritation or injury, consult a physician or podiatrist immediately—meaning, within 24 hours.

Not surprisingly, given all these foot concerns, if you have diabetes, you should see a podiatrist regularly. A podiatrist "plays an integral role" on the treatment team of a person with diabetes, says Robert Katz, DPM, a podiatrist in Bradenton, Florida. "Because diabetes can cause poor bloodflow and nerve damage in lower legs, foot problems are more common in people with diabetes. Any noticeable changes in the feet should be examined by a podiatrist."

The bottom line? If there's any good to be found in diabetes, it's that the condition can motivate you to lead a healthy lifestyle that includes walking regularly. And that means not only better health and greater longevity but also increased enjoyment of life.

CHAPTER 3

THE SECRET OF
A HEALTHY HEART

A gateway sounds like a lovely thing—a trellised arch over a winding path perhaps. But when you're talking about your health, the word has a more sinister implication. A gateway disease is a condition that opens the door to other problems.

Diabetes is a gateway disease because most people with diabetes develop other health problems. For example, they often have high blood pressure and cholesterol, which increase their risk of heart disease and stroke. These risk factors combined with diabetes add up to major problems.

According to the American Diabetes Association, more than 65 percent of people with diabetes die of heart disease or stroke. People with diabetes often have heart attacks earlier in life, and they're more likely to die of them. But by managing their blood pressure and cholesterol, people with diabetes can reduce their risk.

You probably already know that walking and other forms of exercise can reduce the risk of heart disease and stroke. But here's something that may be news to you: Exercising may be *more* important to your heart health than losing weight.

We mention this because weight loss is the reason that many people launch a walking program in the first place. Even if the number on your scale remains unchanged, it doesn't mean that walking isn't doing you any good. It surely is, though in ways you may not be able to see. That's why we always tell people to think in terms of walking for their health, not just for thin thighs and six-pack abs.

Make no mistake: Overweight and obesity are risk factors for a number of ailments, including heart disease. And the more extra pounds you carry, the greater your chances of illness. Doctors have been saying this for years. But newer studies suggest that an active lifestyle, one that may involve regular walking, actually overrides certain risk factors for heart disease, including family history, smoking, and overweight.

FITNESS OUTWEIGHS FATNESS

Leading the way in this groundbreaking research is the famed Cooper Institute for Aerobics Research in Dallas. A team of scientists there, led by Steven Blair, PED, confirmed that fitness is a fabulous overall health protector, even for those of us who are carrying around extra pounds.

For 8 years, Dr. Blair and his colleagues tracked the health status of more than 25,000 men and 7,000 women. The researchers monitored each person's body weight and fitness level (as measured in exercise stress tests) and periodically evaluated blood pressure, blood sugar, and cholesterol levels. They also documented any family history of heart disease as well as smoking habits.

Based on the data they collected, Dr. Blair's team concluded that death rates from all causes, including heart attacks, were lowest among men and women who were moderately to highly fit, regardless of weight (and other risk factors, such as smoking, high cholesterol, high blood pressure, and family history). Sedentary men and women fared worse, regardless of whether they were fat or thin.

DON'T COUNT OUT POUNDS

According to Dr. Blair, it's true that people who are thin generally are more active and fit, and therefore healthier, than people who are overweight. But as his research suggests, thinness without fitness won't protect you against ill-

Proof That Exercise Helps Hearts

In one separate study, 4,000 nurses between ages 40 and 65—all with diabetes—reduced their chances of developing heart disease by 28 percent just by walking regularly. More vigorous exercise lowered their risk another 5 percentage points.

In a separate study involving 5,000 doctors who had experienced heart attacks, those who exercised at least twice a week were 40 percent less likely to die from any cause and 50 percent less likely to die from heart problems.

ness or help you live longer. On the other hand, if you weigh more than you should but you walk or engage in some other physical activity on a regular basis, health-wise you're a step ahead of all those thin couch potatoes.

That's not to say that your weight doesn't matter at all. On the contrary, extra pounds put you at risk for all sorts of health problems, including diabetes and high blood pressure. What you need to keep in mind is that even if you don't lose all the weight you'd like, you still boost your chances of a long, healthy life by being active and fit.

"Virtually every system of your body is affected in some way by regular exercise," Dr. Blair says. "Carbohydrate metabolism improves, and blood sugar levels normalize. There are positive changes in blood fats and blood pressure. Plus, people who exercise regularly simply have stronger hearts."

"Over time, regular exercise slows your resting pulse rate," adds William P. Castelli, MD, medical director of the Framingham Cardiovascular Institute in Framingham, Massachusetts. "The faster your resting pulse, the shorter your life."

To determine your resting pulse rate, check your pulse first thing in the morning, before you even get out of bed. Place two fingers over the carotid artery, located on either side of your neck. Count the beats for 10 seconds, then multiply by 6 for the number of beats per minute. Seventy beats per minute or less is considered healthy. As you become more fit, you may see your resting pulse rate drop. If you get sick or experience some type of stress, your resting pulse rate may jump up.

THE SKINNY ON BELLY FAT

Perhaps the most significant health benefit of regular exercise such as walking is a reduction in intra-abdominal fat. This type of fat collects around internal organs, rather than under the surface of the skin as it does on the hips and thighs. Because of its location, intra-abdominal fat can contribute to serious health problems, including heart disease.

Through studies involving both men and women, researchers at the University of Alabama at Birmingham determined that the primary way exercise lowers heart disease risk is by trimming intra-abdominal fat. In fact, you may be losing this fat even when the number on the scale doesn't change.

That's why Jean-Pierre Després, PhD, director of the Lipid Research Center at Laval University in St. Foy, Quebec, suggests that you trade in your scale for a tape measure. Take an initial measure-

---

Take Symptoms Seriously

If you've been diagnosed with heart disease, high blood pressure, or another heart-related problem, memorize these three warning signs.

- Shortness of breath when you're exercising at your normal level of exertion
- Excessive fatigue, even though you're taking your usual walk
- Any kind of chest discomfort

If you experience any of these symptoms, contact your physician immediately. If your chest pain does not subside with appropriate nitroglycerin therapy, call your local emergency number or have someone take you to the nearest hospital emergency room.

ment of your waist for comparison, then periodically recheck that measurement as you advance in your walking program. Or forget about the tape measure and keep tabs on your waist size using your favorite belt. With every notch you tighten, you'll know you're making progress.

In several studies, Dr. Després found that patients were able to significantly reduce their internal belly fat and almost normalize certain disease risk factors through a combination of regular aerobic exercise and a low-fat diet. The exercise consisted of a 1-hour walk every day.

"Aim for at least 45 minutes, 5 days a week," Dr. Després suggests. "Even 30 minutes a day will help." If you're not up to a brisk pace, walk slower but longer. It's not the speed but the total calories burned that counts.

THE BEST MEDICINE FOR HIGH BLOOD PRESSURE

Here's another way in which exercise may help keep your heart healthy and strong. In combination with proper diet, it appears to lower high blood pressure.

This is important because high blood pressure is one of the many conditions for which doctors frequently prescribe medications. And these medications, like most, can have unwanted side effects.

Yet many people accept prescriptions from their doctors without question. Understandably, they feel uncomfortable challenging the course of treatment recommended by a medical professional—even when other, non-drug options exist. So some doctors get on a sort of medication merry-go-round: They prescribe one blood pressure drug, and if it doesn't work as well as expected, they prescribe another.

When eight prestigious physicians' groups, including the American College of Cardiology and the American College of Preventive Medicine, looked into the treatment of high blood pressure in the United States, they found that doctors favor medication over exercise and diet. Often that's because doctors overlook high blood pressure until medication becomes a necessity.

EARLY INTERVENTION IS BEST

In the United States, an estimated 72 million adults have high blood pressure.

In Step with Stephen Petrakovich

He's on the Road to a Healthier Heart

Steve Petrakovich stood at the bottom of the steep hill at the New Age Health Spa in Neversink, New York, and sighed. The year before, he'd have walked up it easily. But after two heart attacks and two angioplasties, he felt reluctant to even try. While others walked, he climbed into a van, feeling despondent and embarrassed.

At age 56, Steve finally experienced the heart problems that had stalked the rest of his family, killing his father, mother, aunt, and nephew. Angioplasty cleared away the obstructions inside Steve's arteries, but no one seemed interested in how two heart attacks had damaged his emotional well-being, leaving him feeling hopeless, frightened, and alone.

"My doctor focused on my physical symptoms, not my emotional vulnerability," Steve recalls. "At checkups, when he asked me how I felt, I said, 'Fine,' because I figured I *was* fine in the terms he was asking about. I didn't have chest pain. But I felt afraid to do anything, afraid to go places alone, to walk, to drive, to lift anything heavy. I was a wreck inside."

Yet 72 percent of them don't know it. The condition is sly and sneaky. You'll feel no pain or other symptoms as your arteries gum up with fatty debris and your heart strains, weakens, and enlarges.

While blood pressure screenings are routinely performed during visits to doctors' offices, the readings themselves tend to get short shrift. That's because family practitioners and internists, who do those initial screenings, may not have the expertise necessary to properly interpret readings. They may not see high-normal blood pressure as significant, even though it tends to get higher over time. So 5 years down the road, patients who might have controlled their blood pressure through exercise and diet end up on medication instead.

One of the most important changes a

After 3 months of despondency, Steve decided to participate in a Healthy Lifestyles pilot program at the New Age Health Spa. Participants spent a week learning about exercise, healthy eating, and stress reduction. For Steve, it was a real turning point.

"I needed a fresh start. I needed to build confidence in my abilities again, to find new ways to cope with old problems," he explains. "I became more aware that there was a lot that I could gain control over."

Perhaps the most important thing Steve learned was how to take things one step at a time, at his own pace. "The program designer and leader, Bill Bakey, spent one-on-one time with me. He took the time to get into my head and to understand what I was feeling," Steve says. "Bill told me it was okay if I couldn't keep up with everybody else when I walked. He told me to stop and smell the roses instead of worrying about being a burden. He helped me pay attention to my body's signals. If I get tired or feel chest tightness, I can stop, take a few deep breaths, and enjoy the scenery. When I feel rested, I can keep walking. I know that sounds simple, but I really needed someone to take me through that process."

By the time Steve left New Age, he was walking up and down that steep hill twice a day. "And I was beginning to feel like I could get my life back," he adds.

person with even mildly high blood pressure can make is to launch an exercise routine. Aerobic activities such as walking have been shown to lower blood pressure when they're done for 40 minutes at least three times a week. They seem to have the greatest effect on the systolic number in a blood pressure reading. They also tone your heart and other muscles in your body.

Besides regular walking, other lifestyle changes can help lower your blood pressure to where it should be. Your doctor may advise you to quit smoking, restrict your salt intake, and limit your alcohol consumption to no more than two drinks a day.

If you've already been diagnosed with high blood pressure, or if you suspect that you have the condition, see your doctor for a checkup before you begin a walking program. In fact, people older than age 40, regardless of whether they have high blood pressure, should get a physical evaluation before starting an exercise regimen, especially if they have been sedentary for years.

A PRESCRIPTION FOR HEALING YOUR HEART

Even for people who already have heart disease or who have experienced a heart attack or undergone heart surgery, a walking program can work wonders. When you walk regularly, the conditioning effect enhances the pumping ability of your heart, so it's less likely to become overtaxed when you're exerting yourself. In addition, walking may lower your blood pressure, improve your cholesterol profile, and short-circuit the depression that often follows heart surgery.

Because your heart is in a weakened state, you need to be especially careful when starting a walking program. You may have all kinds of questions about what you can and can't do: How fast should I go? Are hills okay? Should I walk after a meal? What about walking when it's hot, cold, or humid? What if I feel pain? Can I safely walk alone?

Since every person's situation is unique, you should discuss these and other questions with your doctor *before* you begin walking. Your doctor may even recommend a specific walking routine for you as part of a comprehensive, supervised cardiac rehabilitation program.

The following general guidelines can help make walking a safe, effective activity while your heart is on the mend. Again, some of these tips may not be appropriate for you, depending on your medical condition. Be sure to review all of them with your doctor.

Make walking part of a plan. Walking is a fabulous activity, but it can't heal your heart on its own. You need to make other lifestyle changes, too. So follow your doctor's orders. If you smoke, quit. Adjust your eating habits. Learn and practice stress-management techniques.

Have your doctor set your limit. One of the most important things for you to do is to identify the point of exertion at which you are putting yourself at risk for a heart attack. Pain may not be the best indicator, because some heart attacks are painless. By using an electrocardiogram (EKG) to track your heart rhythm during an exercise session, your doctor can tell you how hard you can push yourself before you put yourself in danger. He or she can also tell you how to stay within a safe range of exertion.

The challenge is to find a duration that's beneficial but safe. You may have to start at 5 minutes a day. But you'll want to work up to at least 30 minutes a day, at least 5 days a week, with your doctor's approval. Most people can monitor themselves on the basis of how they feel. You may not need to check your pulse or wear complicated pulse-monitoring equipment during workouts.

Maintain a moderate pace. "People should work up to a comfortably brisk pace, where they can still carry on a conversation," says Dean Ornish, MD, author of *Dr. Dean Ornish's Program for Reversing Heart Disease.* His advice may seem simplistic, but it's based on sound, scientific evidence.

You really don't need to worry about going fast enough. The benefits of walking kick in at just 45 percent of your maximum heart rate, so a moderate pace is more than adequate. You do need to be careful about going too fast or too hard, which may do your heart more harm than good. As a rule of thumb,

don't walk so speedily that you become breathless or can't carry on a conversation. If you enjoy intense exercise and want to take up racewalking or speedwalking, be sure to work closely with your doctor.

Disregard distance. Remember, it's how long you walk, not how far, that matters most. The "right" distance is what you can cover comfortably within 30 minutes—and that includes returning to your starting point.

Take it easy after eating. Forgo a brisk walk after a big meal, when blood is being shunted away from your heart and toward your stomach. Allow 2 to 4 hours after eating before engaging in vigorous exercise. A postmeal stroll is okay; in fact, it may help burn calories and enhance digestion. But wait about an hour after eating before heading out, if only to avoid indigestion. (Walking after a light meal generally poses no problems.)

Check out the thermometer. Temperature extremes may put your heart at risk. If it's cold outside, take time to warm up before walking. If it's hot, slow your pace and drink plenty of water en route. Or consider going to the nearest mall when the temperature goes too high or too low.

The Buddy System Packs Triple Benefits

Friends and walking go together like love and marriage. They're all predictors of longer, healthier lives.

Since a Swedish study gave strength to the theory that lack of social support is a risk factor for heart disease in women (other research had already confirmed such a correlation in men), having an exercise buddy would seem to make walking even better for you. How so?

- An exercise buddy provides social support, a predictor of heart health.
- Having a buddy increases the likelihood that you'll stick with your walking program.
- Walking in pairs or with a group makes you less vulnerable to robbery or attack.

While there may be times when you want or need to walk alone, know that stepping out with a partner may provide extra protection for your heart and your health.

The climate-controlled environment is perfect for people with heart problems.

Don't fear going out on your own. Unless you have unstable angina (a condition characterized by severe chest pain) or some other health problem that could trigger a medical emergency, you should be fine to walk by yourself. Teaming up with an exercise buddy, perhaps your spouse or a friend, may make walking more pleasurable and help you stick with your program. But it isn't a medical necessity.

Bag the hand weights. Many experts advise against them. And for people with heart problems, they may pose a serious risk by raising blood pressure.

Stay on level terrain. If a hill is steep enough to make your heart rate climb fast, you should probably avoid it. If that isn't possible, stop as often as necessary during your ascent to rest and allow your heart to recover. Don't press on and tough it out.

Pay attention to how you feel. If you feel as though you're pushing yourself too hard, slow your pace. Or take a brief break, then start walking again. (People with a condition called silent ischemia need to consult their doctors for pulse recommendations. They may be told to wear a heart monitor and to keep their pulses within a specific range when they work out. They can have heart attacks without experiencing pain or even breathlessness.)

You may have heard that stopping too quickly without first cooling down is dangerous for your heart. If you've been walking at a moderate pace, the degree of change should not have any negative effects, such as triggering an irregular heartbeat.

In case of pain, remember the "3 by 5 rule." Keep your nitroglycerin tablets with you at all times. If you experience any chest discomfort while walking, sit down immediately. Then follow what one cardiac rehabilitation center calls the 3 by 5 rule. If your pain doesn't subside within 1 minute, take 1 nitroglycerin tablet under your tongue. Wait 5 minutes. If your pain persists, take another tablet, up to a total of 3 tablets over the course of 15 minutes. You can start walking again as soon as your pain goes away. If it doesn't let up within 15 minutes, call the local number for medical emergencies or have someone drive you to the nearest hospital emergency room.

CHAPTER 4

A SURPRISING RX FOR ARTHRITIS

Although having diabetes doesn't make you susceptible to arthritis, the two conditions do share many characteristics. Also because they are both so common, it's very possible to have them in combination. The older you get, the better your chances of this are because both diabetes and arthritis are age-prevalent. Half of the people with diabetes are older than 60, and arthritis is one of the most common chronic conditions affecting older people. The good news is, walking can be a one-two punch against both conditions.

For years, experts believed that exercise might be bad for people with osteo-arthritis. The most common form of arthritis, it's characterized by the gradual breakdown of cartilage, the spongy material that cushions and protects joints. Over time, this wearing away produces joint stiffness and pain.

Millions of Americans have osteoarthritis, and many of them are understandably reluctant to take the plunge into a program of regular exercise. After all, it's reasonable to assume that walking every day might set the stage for the condition or aggravate existing symptoms.

But now we know that's not the case. In fact, research suggests that walking can prevent or relieve arthritis symptoms. With every step, walking literally cleanses and feeds your foot, knee, and hip joints.

"Cartilage has no blood supply, so it depends on your movement to squeeze out waste products," explains physical therapist Marian Minor, PhD, professor, department chair, and director of Research and Graduate Studies at the University of Missouri School of Health Professions in Columbia. "Between steps, your cartilage sponges up fresh nutrients from the fluid surrounding it."

Imagine that! Every time you walk, it's like taking your joints to the cleaners.

FITNESS FIGHTS WEAR AND TEAR

There is no evidence that exercise is the culprit behind arthritis. On the contrary, exercise may be the perfect salve for arthritic joints.For one study, Stanford University researchers recruited 51 men and women who ran for about 3 hours a week. Some of the runners cut back on their workouts during the study, while the rest either maintained or increased their levels of exercise. When the researchers compared knee x-rays of the study participants taken over a 2-year period, they found no significant differences in the number of tiny, lumpy joint growths that are a telltale sign of osteoarthritis.

Study author James Fries, MD, emeritus professor of medicine at Stanford University, says that in 25 years of working with runners who log a whopping 40

Expand Your Exercise Horizons

For people with arthritis, an activity such as yoga, tai chi, or water therapy can be a great complement to walking. The exercises gently move your joints through their full range of motion, so you don't feel stiff and sore when you walk.

Water therapy, in particular, has been popular as an arthritis treatment for many years. Exercising in water helps take some of the pressure off aching joints. In addition, the warmth of the water may have a relaxing effect.

In one study, British researchers had 35 people with arthritis move around in a tub of hot water for 30 minutes twice a week. After 4 weeks, the participants reported that their joints felt less stiff. And the effect lasted for months.

Some people with arthritis start their walking programs in the pool, then move onto dry land as they get stronger and more flexible. But they still love their water workouts.

> ## Quick Tip
>
> If you're concerned that a long workout may take you too far from home—and that you'll be hurting too much for the return trip—choose a short, circular route around your neighborhood. You can still walk for 30 minutes, but you'll never be more than a block away from home.

to 100 miles a week, he found that they're better off—much better off—than their couch-potato counterparts. "You'd expect the x-rays of runners to be worse than those of nonrunners," he says. "But they're not. They're exactly the same. Yet runners have *less* pain and disability than people who are sedentary."

And if running doesn't accelerate the deterioration of joints, walking certainly won't. That should warm you up to the idea of starting a walking program.

STRATEGIES FOR PAIN-FREE PERAMBULATION

If you have osteoarthritis and you haven't been exercising regularly, Dr. Minor recommends that you start out by walking at a moderate intensity 4 to 6 days a week.

(Moderate intensity means that you should be able to sing a song as you go along, without becoming breathless.) Your goal is to accumulate at least 30 minutes of exercise a day, every day. Of course, you'll have to work up to that. In the beginning, you may want to break down those 30 minutes into 10-minute segments, spread over the course of a day.

Each time you walk for 30 minutes, spend the first 5 to 10 warming up with an easy stroll. Once you're warmed up, take time to stretch. (You can use the Dynamic Body Exercises described in Chapter 34.) Stretching creates space in your joints, which eases discomfort. Then you're ready to pick up your stride until you reach a comfortable pace. As you near the end of your workout, slow your pace a bit to cool down. If you have time, stretch again.

EXTRA HELP FOR HURTING KNEES

If walking proves to be more of a pain than you can tolerate, don't pack up your walking shoes. Give your joints time to adjust. You may need to take an over-the-counter or prescription pain reliever to ease any discomfort. Ask your doctor to recommend a brand and dosage.

In addition, some of these strategies may help keep your walks pain free.

Experiment with magnets. Although there's no conclusive scientific evidence that magnets help reduce pain, many people, including lots of athletes, swear by them. Just remember, the kind that you stick on your refrigerator won't do the job. Therapeutic magnets, which are available in many drugstores and department stores, are specially designed and have greater strength than ordinary household magnets.

Pick up some walking sticks. Using two walking sticks, held like cross-country ski poles, can take pressure off your knee joints. As a bonus, doing this increases your calorie burn and helps build your upper-body strength. (For more information on walking with poles, see page 131.)

Unload the excess baggage. Because of your body's mechanics, every extra pound of body weight feels like another 8 to 10 pounds to your hips, knees, and ankles. So lose 5 pounds of fat, and you gain 50 pounds' worth of pain relief.

Sign up for a class. The Arthritis Foundation offers an Arthritis Self-Help Program at various locations across the United States that, among other things, shows participants how to exercise properly. In one study, people who enrolled in the class reported an 18 percent reduction in their pain. The 6-week course costs between $25 and $50. For more information, visit the Arthritis Foundation's Web site, www.arthritis.org.

CHAPTER 5

GOOD NEWS FOR BAD BACKS

What do diabetes and bad backs have in common? Obesity for one: Almost 90 percent of people with diabetes are overweight, and according to some estimates almost half of the people with back pain are obese. Also by the sheer numbers of people who have diabetes (7 percent of Americans) and back problems (10 percent of Americans), very likely another thing diabetes and bad backs have in common is you.

Time was when an aching back could lay you up for days, if not weeks. But not anymore. While a day or two of bed rest might be part of your pain relief prescription, most doctors want you to get on your feet as soon as you can. And often they recommend walking to help you do it.

In fact, walking is so good for bad backs that it has become an integral part of the treatment programs at most back-pain clinics. It strengthens the muscles that support good posture and triggers the release of chemicals called endorphins, which subdue pain and encourage relaxation. What's more, it conditions and tones your entire body.

People who have consistent walking programs tend to recover faster from back injuries than those who don't. Plus, walking helps them keep their weight in check, making them less likely to develop back pain in the first place. So if you're not yet a walker, you have another reason to become one.

Of course, even the fittest among us are vulnerable to back injury—whether from lifting a heavy object improperly, straining to retrieve a book from a too high shelf, playing 36 holes of golf, or coping with a stressful situation that sends back muscles into painful spasms.

With proper care, you can beat back pain. And walking has everything to do with your recovery.

GIVE YOUR BACK A BREAK

When you hurt your back, the first decision you must make is whether or not you need medical attention. Get yourself to your doctor or the nearest hospital emergency room if you experience any of the following:

- Your pain is so intense that you can't move around at all.
- You lose control of your bladder or bowels.
- Your pain is accompanied by fever, nausea or vomiting, sweating, or discomfort when urinating.
- Your pain is associated with some kind of trauma, such as a car accident.
- Your leg or foot feels numb or tingly.
- Your pain radiates to your buttock, thigh, or leg.

If you have none of the symptoms above, then you're probably dealing with garden-variety back muscle spasms. In

that case, you're a good candidate for self-care.

Depending on the severity of your pain, you may want to take it easy until you feel better. Rest is a good way to start off your recovery—as long as you limit it to a day or two, as mentioned earlier.

Lie down with your knees bent and your back flat. Put a pillow or towel under your knees if you need to. This keeps you from straining your back muscles. To pass the time, you can read, watch television, listen to music, or talk on the telephone. Whatever you do, avoid sitting in a chair, because that position is extremely hard on your back muscles. You may even want to eat standing up.

And remember: Rest means just that. If your dry cleaning is waiting to be picked up or your dog needs to go for a walk, ask someone else to do it. Refrain from lifting heavy objects. Being a martyr is noble, but it won't help your back heal.

While you're on the mend, you can take an over-the-counter anti-inflammatory, such as aspirin or ibuprofen, to help relieve pain and reduce any swelling. You can also apply ice to the sore spot. Wrap an ice pack in a towel, hold it against the affected area for 20 minutes, then take it off for 40 minutes before repeating.

> ## Quick Tip
>
> When a back injury puts you to bed for a day or two, take care whenever you get up. Support yourself by rolling onto your side and pushing yourself up with your arms. This minimizes strain on your back muscles.

Most doctors recommend using ice for the first 48 hours, then switching to heat. A warm to comfortably hot shower may do the trick.

BEGIN WALKING WITH BABY STEPS

During those first couple of days after you hurt your back, you can afford to put your walking program on hold. Such a short break won't cause you to lose muscle tone or aerobic conditioning. At the same time, don't expect to walk a 5-K as soon as your ache quiets down.

Once you're ready to start moving around again, you need to spend a few days just getting used to being on your feet. Your first goal is to sit or stand comfortably for 20 minutes. At that point, you're ready to take a short stroll.

Put on the most comfortable and supportive walking shoes that you own. Then choose a route that's easy and on level ground. (Hills make you lean forward, which puts strain on your lower back.) Walk around the outside of your house, out to your mailbox, or to the end of your block and back. Just keep it short.

Some people find that they have trouble standing completely straight when they're first getting back on their feet. If this happens to you, don't be too concerned. You'll likely be able to straighten up as you walk. Walking boosts your circulation, which may relax your back muscles.

On the other hand, if you feel tension building in your upper back as you walk, it may be because you're subconsciously trying to protect your lower back. In that case, consider wearing a lumbar support. It's a stretchy belt that wraps around your waist to relieve stress on your lower-back muscles.

As your back gets better, you may be able to take several short walks over the course of a day, with long periods of rest in between. This helps keep your back limber without straining it.

When you feel ready, you want to gradually increase the duration of your walks. You can expect to feel some pain initially. The question is, how much is too much? It's really a matter of trial and error. You may hurt for a few minutes, then limber up as you go along and feel fine the rest of the way. That's okay. But if your pain starts while you're walking and lingers for hours afterward, you're probably pushing yourself too hard too soon. You need to go a little easier your next time out.

At this stage, it's a good idea to stick with walking routes that continually take you past your door. That way, when the pain doesn't go away, you can head for home and lie down. The last thing you want to do now is reinjure yourself.

What if you can't walk without pain, but you can't sit still? Consider moving your walking workout to a heated pool at a gym or the local YMCA. The water supports your weight, minimizing demands on your back muscles. And the heat soothes any soreness.

Another option is to pedal a stationary cycle. Just be sure to sit in a position that feels comfortable for you.

POSTURE MAKES PERFECT

While walking is an important part of any back-care program, it can actually aggravate back pain if it's done with poor posture. Be careful not to hang your head, hunch over, or lean forward, all of which can push your body out of alignment.

People who are swaybacked (a condition called *lordosis*) or who have a flat lumbar curve in the lower back are especially vulnerable to back trouble. They may feel more pain, not less, when they take long walks because of the pressure put on the spine.

If you want a strong, healthy back that can support you for miles and miles, practicing good posture is essential. We'll discuss body position and movement in greater detail in Part VII. But for now, these tips can help you keep your back pain free while walking.

- Think tall. That old image of a wire attached to the top of your head, pulling it upward, works well.
- Keep your shoulders relaxed rather than throwing them back military-style.
- Imagine that your pelvic bone is tilting up and in toward your navel, creating a slight pelvic tilt.

- Allow your spine to move from side to side as you step from one foot to the other. Don't stiffen your lower back.
- Use short strides, not long ones. The farther you reach forward, the greater the impact on your spine.

STOP PAIN BY STRETCHING

Besides practicing good posture, one of the easiest ways to prevent back pain while walking is by stretching. When your muscles are tight, they can actually constrict blood vessels and impede circulation. And without good circulation, you're more vulnerable to muscle spasms and back injury.

In Part VII, you'll learn stretching exercises that target muscles in your calves, shins, thighs, buttocks, and lower back—all of which support your every step. The following stretches are designed specifically for people with chronic back pain. Do 10 repetitions of each stretch every day. If your pain worsens, discontinue the exercises and see your doctor.

PARTIAL SITUP

LIE on your back with your knees bent and your feet flat on the floor. Position your hands behind your head. Lift your shoulders off the floor, hold for 5 seconds, and lower.

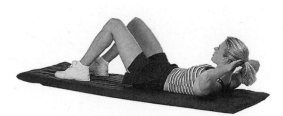

PELVIC LIFT

LIE on your back with your knees bent, your feet flat on the floor, and your hands behind your head. Lift your pelvis off the floor. Extend your right leg so that it's at a 45-degree angle to the floor. Be sure to keep your midback on the floor. Hold for 5 seconds, then lower. Repeat with your left leg.

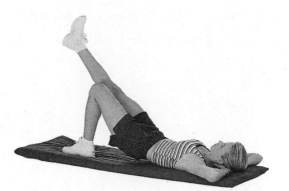

TABLE POSE

GET down on all fours. Lift your left arm and right leg so that they're in line with your spine. Hold for 5 seconds, then lower. Repeat with your right arm and left leg.

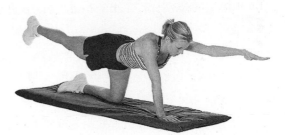

CHAPTER 6

A STEP AHEAD OF STRESS

What makes you want to walk?

When we posed that question to *Prevention* magazine readers who walk a few years back, we expected to get answers like "to lose weight" and "to get in shape." But we were delighted by the number of people who commented on walking's emotional benefits, and in particular on its ability to relieve stress.

Aerobic exercise of any kind has the power to calm jangled nerves and improve bad moods. And when it's done every day, it can enhance self-esteem and combat depression. Indeed, research has shown that a brisk 20- to 30-minute walk can have the same calming effect as a mild tranquilizer.

Why is walking—or any physical activity, for that matter—such a potent stress reducer? Many experts cite its ability to trigger the release of endorphins, potent brain chemicals that relieve pain and stimulate relaxation. Simply put, the higher your level of endorphins, the greater your sense of calm and well-being. No wonder walking can make you feel so good.

STROLL TOWARD RELAXATION

To reap the stress-busting benefits of walking, you don't need to pound the pavement or push yourself really hard. In fact, at least one study has shown that a comfortable stroll can be just as effective as a brisk walk. The key is to use your mind while you're moving your body.

For the study, researchers recruited 135 volunteers and divided them into five groups. Three of the groups took up walking—one at a brisk pace, the other two at a low-intensity pace. The fourth group practiced mindful exercise, which is based on the principles and movements of tai chi. The fifth group served as controls—meaning, they were asked not to change anything about their lives.

In addition, one of the groups assigned to walk at a low-intensity pace learned a simple meditation technique to practice while exercising. All they had to do was pay attention to their footsteps, counting "one, two, one, two" and visualizing each number in their minds as they went along. If they found their thoughts drifting to other matters, they simply said, "Oh, well," and resumed counting their footsteps.

The combination of meditating and low-intensity walking produced dramatic results, according to cardiologist James Rippe, MD, founder and director of the Rippe Lifestyle Institute, who has written several books on the health benefits of walking.

A Tangled Web: The Diabetes-Stress Connection

"Diabetes can cause stress, and stress can affect diabetes," says Kashif Munir, MD, an endocrinologist and medical director of the Joslin Diabetes Center at Baltimore Washington Medical Center in Glen Burnie, Maryland. "Diabetes puts a lot of burden on a person. It's a disease that requires a lot of lifestyle changes. You have to monitor your blood sugar, change your diet, and exercise. All of this leads to stress. Patients sometimes say, 'It's too much for me.'"

To make matters worse, stress in turn affects blood sugar. "Stress hormones, such as cortisol and catecholamines, counteract the effects of insulin, which can make your blood sugar levels go up," says Dr. Munir. "I know a man with diabetes who uses a continuous glucose monitor, which checks his blood sugar levels every 5 minutes. One day he told me that when he was driving toward the DC Beltway, he saw his blood sugar level going up and up. He could see in real time what stress was doing to his blood sugar."

Why Walking Works

The verdict is in: Walking is a top-notch stress-buster. That's what folks told us when we posted an informal survey about stress on our Web site, www.prevention.com.

Whenever you're feeling too overwhelmed to work out, take a moment to read through the following real-life testimonials on the benefits of walking. We bet you'll be instantly inspired to slip on your walking shoes and head out.

"I've learned that stress is energy. I have to deal with it physically, and walking is the best approach for me. I use a treadmill about 95 percent of the time, and nothing feels better than hopping on, working up a good sweat, and talking to myself. Sometimes I drive to a nearby small town, go for a walk, and have a nice long chat with myself. Before I know it, I've covered 3 or 4 miles, and I've gotten to know myself better!"

"Walking definitely calms me down. It helps me connect with the natural world in all the different seasons. I usually walk at night, after dinner. All the tensions of the day melt away, plus I like moving after I've eaten a big meal. Walking allows me to let my mind wander. My thoughts become more random, and I notice how the moonlight colors a tree. Sometimes I window-shop downtown. At bedtime, I often write about what I feel or see on my evening stroll."

"I commute 2 hours to and from work each day. I am so stressed by the time I get home, the first thing I do is grab an apple or pretzels and my walking

During the 16 weeks of the study, the people who meditated while they walked reported decreases in anxiety, along with fewer negative and more positive feelings about themselves. In fact, the ben-efits were equal to those associated with brisk walking. Even better, they were evident after just one session, and they lasted for the duration of the study.

By comparison, the people who walked

shoes. I can usually convince my dad to come with me. All I need is a good, brisk 35- to 40-minute walk, and I feel great again."

"Walking at a fast pace really seems to relieve my stress. The first few minutes feel stressful. But after my body gets going, I feel a burst of energy, and the tension falls away. It's worth the effort!"

"Walking seems to make everything about me better. I'm much more calm and in control than when I started my program 7 months ago. Other people have noticed the changes in my personality as well as the physical changes!"

"Walking is more than a healthy habit. It is mentally therapeutic. Walking helped me through a traumatic divorce and through writer's block. Every day, it improves my state of mind."

"Being outdoors for 30 to 60 minutes, walking, clears my head and lets me focus on things that are really important rather than on the petty things that have annoyed me during the day. Walking frees pent-up energy that I've had to hold back at work. And I feel terrific when I'm done!"

"Walking is the only way I know to calm my mind. I have a good life, but with a home, three daughters, and a husband with multiple sclerosis, it sometimes gets tough to keep my head clear. I've tried other types of exercise, but this is what works for me!"

"When I first started walking, it was slow going. But eventually, I could do 2 miles in 30 minutes. Between exercising daily and making some changes in my diet, I have lowered my cholesterol by 65 points, reduced my blood pressure, and lost 45 pounds. I know that this has saved my life."

at a low-intensity pace but didn't meditate showed no improvements until the 14th week, and even then, the effects weren't as significant. On the other hand, the people who engaged in mindful exercise experienced results that were very similar to those reported by the walking-plus-meditation group, suggesting that other mental techniques could yield stress-busting benefits.

According to Dr. Rippe, one of the most impressive findings from this research is the immediacy with which walking can relieve stress. The study also provided good news for people who aren't able to engage in high-intensity exercise: They can capitalize on walking's de-stressing effects just by practicing meditation or another mental technique during their strolls. And for people who find relaxation exercises tedious or boring, the study proved that a brisk walk can do just as good a job of short-circuiting stress.

KEEP WALKING . . . NO MATTER WHAT

By participating in a regular walking program, you can offset the long-term health implications of stress—and there are many. Research has linked stress to a host of physical ills, from back pain and stomach upset to high

In Step with Melissa and Merle Knapp

Walking Keeps Them Worry Free

When a personal crisis turned their world upside down, Melissa and Merle Knapp took up walking to help them cope. It turned out to be their salvation.

"My husband and I weren't always walkers," Melissa explains. "He felt that walking was no fun and not worth his time."

That was before financial disaster struck. Suddenly, the Knapps found themselves faced with the possibility of losing their home—something they had worked so long and hard for. The strain became almost too much to bear.

"Anyone who has endured an emotional trauma knows that it can be devastating to the body as well as to the mind," Melissa says. "The stress felt like tentacles squeezing my heart. I had constant headaches. And my husband lost his appetite."

Then one morning, Merle asked Melissa if she wanted to go for a walk, explaining that he had to do something to release his tension. Melissa agreed,

blood pressure and heart disease.

Of course, when you're under pressure, whatever its source, going for a walk may be the last thing on your mind. You're not the only one who feels that way. When researchers tracked the exercise habits of 82 women for 8 weeks, they found that the women worked out less often during weeks that were filled with stressful events. At those times, exercise was "just one more thing to do."

When walking starts to feel like a stress *producer* instead of a stress reducer, making some adjustments in your workout can help. Here's what to do.

Adopt the right attitude. Tell yourself that taking a walk will help you accomplish more on your "to do" list. Exercise makes you feel better and think more clearly, so you become more productive.

Aim for the a.m. Walking first thing in the morning, before anyone else is out and about, gives you an opportunity to focus on yourself, says Suki

suggesting that they go to a park that was just far enough from home to seem new to them.

Once there, they found a 2.8-mile loop with a breathtaking view of Washington's Puget Sound. The path was beautiful, with a varied terrain.

"That very first walk performed magic," Melissa recalls. "I don't know whether it was the soothing colors of nature or the rhythm of walking, but I do know that we felt better, even though our problems hadn't changed." They decided to walk the trail every day.

Besides relieving their tension and taking their minds off their financial situation, walking gave the Knapps an opportunity to connect with the world around them. They came to recognize other regular walkers on the path, and they seemed like kindred spirits. "It felt good to smile and say, 'How are you today?'" Melissa says. "We hadn't done much smiling for a while."

These days, the Knapps are happy to report that their finances have improved, and their stress is under control. "And we still walk every day," Melissa says.

Munsell, PhD, director of the Dynamic Health and Fitness Institute in San Anselmo, California. "When my day looks hectic, with lots of decisions ahead, an early-morning walk brings answers and clarity," she notes.

Seek out new scenery. Choose a walking route that takes you down quiet streets or through a beautiful park. The more appealing your surroundings, the calmer you'll feel. Walking on busy streets, in unsafe neighborhoods, or after dark only adds to your stress.

Slow your pace. Pushing yourself to go faster or farther only adds to your stress. During tense times, keep your walks leisurely.

Break up your workout. If your schedule is so busy that you can't find one chunk of time for your walk, take advantage of spare minutes throughout the day. Head outdoors for a stroll before or after lunch or between appointments. Even 5 minutes of walking is enough to recharge your batteries.

TURN YOUR BACK ON TENSION

While maintaining a regular walking program can counteract the physical effects of stress, you don't have to wait until your nerves are in knots to let walking work its magic. Here are some ways that you can incorporate walking into your daily routine—and derail stress before it gets the best of you.

Opt for a 10-minute trot. At work, pass up the break-time doughnut and coffee and go for a walk instead. Research has shown that walking briskly can give you a bigger energy boost than eating a sugary snack. If you're able to go outside, the fresh air and sunshine can clear out those mental cobwebs and brighten your mood. If you can't get out, cruise the hallways of your workplace or climb a flight of stairs. You'll arrive back in your work area refreshed and ready to concentrate.

Take the show on the road. Nervous about a meeting with your boss, a co-worker, or a client? Suggest making it a walk-and-talk session. Walking can relieve your tension and anxiety, so you're more at ease. And you're not face-to-face with the other person, so you avoid the constant eye contact that can be stressful in itself, especially if the topic of your conversation is upsetting or unpleasant.

Walk away from a dilemma. Sometimes you're faced with a knotty problem that can leave you feeling knotted up as well. That's when thinking less and moving more can be a real asset. Drop what you're doing and take a stress-free stroll, letting your mind wander as you do. By the time you return to face the problem at hand, the answer that you were racking your brain for may seem obvious.

Use your feet to run errands. It's an all-too-familiar scenario: You hop in your car early Saturday morning and head for the bank or the drugstore, hoping to beat the long lines. Instead, you spend a half hour circling your destination in search of a parking space—and by the time you find one, you're fit to be tied. Next time, try leaving your car at home and doing your errands on foot. You'll avoid the aggravation of clogged streets and parking lots, and you may even save time.

Park prudently. Cars pulling in and out, shopping carts rolling about, and people rushing in every direction—a parking lot seems like an accident waiting to happen. If you must drive in one, do what you can to keep yourself out of the fray. Park as far from other cars and the entrance as you can. If you can safely do so, walk around the perimeter of the parking lot before heading inside. Then you can face the crowds without feeling frazzled.

CHAPTER 7

THE PIONEERING PROS OF WALKING

When a salesman is trying to sell you a new car, you're more likely to believe what he's saying if he drives the same make that he's pitching to you. After all, who wants to buy a Chevy from a guy who tools around town in a Toyota?

Likewise, when your doctor tells you that you need to exercise, you're more inclined to heed his advice if he's following it himself. These days, he probably is.

Now more than ever, physicians and other health professionals are practicing what they prescribe, especially in terms of exercise. And often their activity of choice is walking.

Over the years, we've been fortunate enough to meet many of these health practitioners and hear their inspiring stories. Now we'd like to share a few of those stories with you. Read them and see if you aren't just a bit more convinced that walking can do wonders for your health and well-being.

HELPING A CITY SLIM DOWN

Herman Frankel, MD, founder of the Portland Health Institute in Portland, Oregon, "discovered" walking some 25 years ago. Back then, he was a busy pediatrician with an especially stressful schedule in a hospital nursery.

At the end of one particularly rough day, Dr. Frankel decided to take a walk. He felt so much better that he vowed to make walking part of his routine.

Every morning before he went to the hospital, he walked for 45 minutes. Within a year—without making any other changes in his lifestyle—he lost 15 pounds.

The experience piqued Dr. Frankel's interest in the effects of low-intensity exercise on body composition. He had always believed that only heart-pounding, sweat-producing workouts could provide any benefit. Now he had firsthand evidence that walking at a moderate pace could burn fat.

Five years later, he would put his theory to the test in a very public arena. He and the staff of a Portland-based television show launched a program called "Fight against Fat." Six female volunteers, chosen from among hundreds, went on a weight reduction plan that emphasized a low-fat diet and regular walking. The women appeared on the TV show once a month to share their experiences with viewers. In turn, viewers could write to the show for self-help packets that included graphs for charting their own daily walks. By the time the program ended, all six women—and hundreds of people who had watched their progress—had lost weight.

"Fight against Fat" was considered such a success that it won the United States Secretary of Health and Human Services Award for Excellence in Community Health Promotion and Disease Prevention. As for Dr. Frankel, he continued his personal regimen of walking regularly and eating healthfully. The last time we spoke with him, his weight was holding steady, at just 5 pounds more than his weight at age 26, when he was a national-level volleyball player.

FITNESS IS HIS PRESCRIPTION

When we interviewed Neil Block, MD, a family physician from Orangeburg, New York, he told us that he had taken up walking to ease his back pain and maintain his weight. He figured that the regular workouts would help fend off heart disease, too, a healthy bonus. He managed to work up to a speedy 12-minute-per-mile pace, exercising for 40 to 60 minutes, three or four times a week.

Because of his busy schedule, Dr. Block fit in his walks whenever he could—even if it was just before bedtime. Some people say that late-night workouts overstimulate them and keep them awake. But Dr. Block found that he not only slept very well but also fell asleep faster.

In his practice, he advised almost all of his patients to walk, even one gentleman with emphysema who had been relying on others to drive him everywhere. Eventually, this man was able to walk to stores and to the library on his own. "You can't grow new air sacs [in your lungs], but you can make sure that your diaphragm and other muscles that support respiration are strong," Dr. Block explained.

To help his patients follow his walking prescription, Dr. Block sometimes walked with them—around a nearby lake in the summer, at a local mall or health club in the winter. "Walking is part of a healthy lifestyle," he observed. "My business card says, 'Family Practice—Lifestyle Changes.' Correct habits create health. Walking creates health."

SETTING AN EXAMPLE THROUGH EXERCISE

You might say that Ross Stryker, DDS, was an orthodontist with a mission. He had seen so many out-of-shape adolescents in his Missouri dental practice that he planned an 8-day walk to celebrate his personal commitment to fitness (and to have some fun). On November 8, 1998, he set out on a 250-mile journey along the Katy Trail, which runs from Clinton to St. Charles, Missouri.

The Katy Trail is a converted railroad bed, perhaps the longest and flattest in the country. Dr. Stryker arranged to stay at bed-and-breakfasts along the way. His wife, Mary, sent care packages to the innkeepers, so he could walk relatively unencumbered. "Although I was trying to make a statement about the importance of exercise, such as walking, mostly I just enjoyed myself!" he says.

During his walk, Dr. Stryker wore a bright orange vest with flashing lights. Hunting season had arrived, and lots of hunters were out early in the morning. "I would start walking at 6:30 a.m. in total darkness," he recalls. "Slowly, the sun would come up—first a small hint of light, then a glow in the clouds on the horizon. It was the perfect time of day for me, and a great time to spot wildlife on the move."

A dedicated 50-mile-a-week walker, Dr. Stryker displays mementos from his Katy Trail trek in his office to generate interest among his patients. He hopes that they'll be motivated to take up walking and make it a lifelong activity.

For more information on the Katy Trail—including maps, mileage charts, and more—visit the Bike Katy Trail Web site at www.bikekatytrail.com.

PART II

ARE YOU
READY TO WALK?

CHAPTER 8

SHOES: THE FACTS ABOUT FIT

If you are going to be a walker, especially if you have diabetes, you need one very important piece of equipment. Well, actually two: a pair of good walking shoes. They will be your best walking buddies—for 6 months to a year, anyway. So choose them with care. And when you find that perfect-fitting style, stay with it.

There is a shoe out there for everybody—or, more precisely, for every foot. You just need to know a few facts so that you can get the right fit. An expensive shoe that's the wrong size or shape won't serve you as well as a moderately priced shoe that accommodates the contours of your foot, bending where your foot bends and giving your toes ample wiggle room.

Once you find a great pair of walking shoes and you discover what real comfort feels like, you may not want to subject your feet to anything else. The best news is that finding a pair of shoes that is comfortable as well as stylish has gotten a lot easier. More and more footwear manufacturers are realizing that many consumers will no longer sacrifice comfort and foot health for fashion.

So how do you find the perfect match for your feet? Let's get down to some shoe-buying basics.

LEARN THE LINGO

Before you go shoe shopping, take a few minutes to familiarize yourself with the following terms. The salesperson you deal with should understand

Time to Buy New Shoes

To keep your feet, ankles, knees, and lower back healthy and injury free, replace your walking shoes every 500 to 700 miles. Beyond that distance, even if the shoes don't look worn-out, their shock-absorbing capacity is no longer as good as it used to be.

If you're not sure how long you've had your current pair of shoes, set them on a table and examine them from the heel. Does the heel show any signs of wear? Does the upper look as though it has been pushed toward one side by your foot? Then it's definitely time to invest in a new pair.

On the day of your purchase, mark the date inside your shoes with a permanent marker, or in your logbook. Then, using your logbook, you'll be able to track your mileage, so you'll know when you need a new pair. Or if you consistently walk, say, 3 miles for 5 days a week (or 15 miles per week), you can mark the "expiration date" of your current shoes on your calendar.

People with diabetes should have two pairs of walking shoes on hand rather than just one. That way, you can allow each pair to dry out completely after each use. Walking in wet shoes is like putting out a welcome sign for blisters and athlete's foot, both of which are dangerous for people with diabetes. Dry shoes also minimize foot odor and create a less-hospitable environment for bacteria. Plus, when you buy a new pair, you can switch between them and an old pair, one that has already formed to your feet. Your feet will appreciate your consideration.

this terminology, too. It can make a world of difference in the quality and fit of the shoe you take home.

EVA: A shock-absorbing foam that's soft, light, and flexible, EVA is found in the soles of many good walking shoes. It compresses on long walks but springs back after a day of rest. Some shoes have dual-density EVA, which simply means that the material has two different compression rates.

Heel-strike: This is the point where your heel makes contact with the ground if you're using proper walking technique. You need to consider heel-strike when selecting a shoe, because your heel takes a pounding with each step—and that may happen thousands of times when you're out walking. Look for a shoe that provides stability, with a slightly beveled heel and plenty of cushioning.

Last: This is the mold on which a shoe is formed. The last—and, therefore, the bottom of the shoe—can be straight, semi-curved, or curved. For a good fit, make sure that the shape of your shoe matches the shape of your foot. (We'll help you determine the shape of your foot in the next section.)

Medial support: Sounds fancy, but don't let the term confuse you. It simply means arch support.

Overpronation: This means that your ankle rolls inward when you're walking, which puts way too much pressure on your arch and nearby ligaments and tissues. Over time, overpronation can lead to heel pain and other problems. A good shoe supports and stabilizes your ankle so that it doesn't roll inward.

Sockliner: Every good shoe has one of these inserts, which cushions and protects your foot from the shoe's "guts." Without a sockliner, you would feel stitching or little lumps of glue when you walk.

Toebox: This is the part of a shoe that encases your piggies. It should be roomy, both in width and in height. And it should somewhat resemble the toe-end of your foot. No more pointy toes.

SIZE MATTERS— BUT THAT'S NOT ALL

To ensure that your shoes fit well, you need to learn a bit more about your feet. What we're going to explain now may surprise even some shoe salespeople. But that's okay. Armed with this information, you can help yourself.

For a shoe to fit properly, it has to match your foot type—that is, its flexibility—and curvature. You can easily

---

Quick Tip

If you can't spread your toes inside your walking shoes, then you need wider shoes. A too small toebox results in the overuse or underuse of certain bones, muscles, tendons, and ligaments. Your entire body must compensate for that.

assess these characteristics on your own in a few simple steps.

Flexibility refers to whether your foot is rigid, neutral, or flexible. To find out, do the following:

1. Sit in a chair, with one foot resting across the opposite knee. Measure the elevated foot from the heel to the tip of the longest toe (usually your big toe) by holding a ruler against the sole. Be careful not to press on the ruler, as that will skew the measurement. Write down the number, then do the same with your other foot.

2. Lay the ruler on the floor and stand on it with one foot. Measure from the heel to the tip of the longest toe. Write down the number, then switch feet and repeat.

3. Determine your foot type based on these descriptions.
    - If the measurements taken when seated and when standing are about the same, your feet are rigid.
    - If the measurements differ by about $1/8$ inch, your feet are neutral.
    - If the measurements differ by about $1/4$ inch, your feet are flexible.

Now that you know your foot type, you're ready to determine your foot curvature—that is, whether your foot is straight, semi-curved, or curved. Here's what to do.

1. Sit in a chair, with a piece of paper on the floor in front of you.

2. Put your left foot on the paper so that it's pointed straight ahead. Lift your toes upward to stabilize the shape of your foot.

3. Either by yourself or with someone's help, trace the outline of your foot on the paper.

4. Pick up the paper and fold the outline of your foot in half, bringing the heel up over the toe. Then fold the heel-end back down, so the heel is visible.

5. Compare your outline to the three below. Select the one that matches yours.

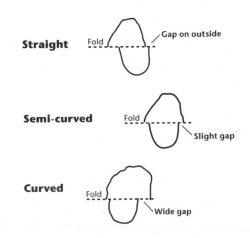

THE RIGHT SHOE FOR YOUR TYPE

Armed with your foot type and curvature, you're ready to do some shoe shopping. Give the information to a knowledgeable shoe salesperson, who should be able to recommend just the right shoe for your foot. Or you can do the matching-up yourself.

To find a shoe that has the proper curvature, or last, cut out the foot outline that you traced and take it with you when you go shopping. Hold the outline against the bottom of each shoe that you like. You'll be able to tell which shoe is going to fit your foot comfortably. (You'll also be able to check to see whether a shoe is long enough and wide enough for you.)

To make sure that a shoe is appropriate for your foot type, look for the following features.

Rigid: Rigid feet are very stiff and tend to have high arches. They're stable, but they don't handle impact well. For this foot type, you need a shoe that is very well-cushioned, because your arch is not going to flex and provide much cushioning for you. You also need an upper that has a lot of volume, or space, to accommodate your high instep. You may have tight Achilles tendons (at the backs of your ankles), so you'll want your shoe to have a bit of a heel. Most rigid feet are curved, so a shoe with a curved last will fit better.

Neutral: This foot type is the easiest to fit. A neutral foot has normal mobility, which means it lengthens or spreads about half a shoe size when bearing weight (when you stand up, for example). It absorbs shock well and has good stability. You can get by with less support, although a little extra won't hurt either. For a neutral foot, a shoe with a semi-curved last should fit well.

Flexible: Of the three foot types, flexible feet are the most complicated and most

Quick Tip

Ask other walkers or, better yet, runners where they buy their shoes. Runners often know the best stores. Their feet take a lot of abuse, so if they want to run for long, they need really great-fitting shoes.

The Great Shoe Debate

For years, controversy has raged over whether running shoes are acceptable for walkers. Remember, running shoes came first. Before 1986, you couldn't even buy walking shoes. Stores carried "comfort shoes" or canvas shoes with rubber soles, what baby boomers know as sneakers.

Walking shoes have come a long way since then. They've gotten a lot better. At first, they looked like nurses' shoes or orthopedic shoes. Now they're engineered with just as much technical know-how as running shoes, and they have lots of product testing behind them.

Running requires far more cushioning and stability than walking, but that doesn't mean you can't wear running shoes for walking. The fit is what counts.

Running shoes tend to be flashier than walking shoes in design and color. And they're usually more plentiful than walking shoes, so you have more brands and styles to choose from. On the downside, running shoes tend to have thicker soles

difficult to fit. They absorb shock well because they are so mobile, but that mobility tends to make them unstable. They change one whole size when bearing weight. They also tend to be flat and have a low instep. If you have flexible feet, look for shoes with low volume—meaning, little distance from the laces to the soles. You don't need a lot of cushioning, but you do need a lot of support. You also need a low heel, which will do a better job of stabilizing your foot. You may feel most comfortable in a shoe with a straight last because your foot tends to flatten and straighten out when you walk.

BRANDS THAT MEASURE UP

As we said before, there is a shoe out there for every foot. So don't settle for less than a perfect fit. Expect to pay between $55 and $100 for a good-quality, good-fitting pair of walking shoes. If the price seems high, consider the cost of an appointment with a podiatrist or ortho-

than walking shoes. They'll make you taller, but they'll also make you more prone to tripping. So be careful!

The bottom line: Walking shoes are specifically designed to help propel you through the heel-toe motion of the proper walking technique. While runners land flat-footed, walkers land on their heels. So the heels of walking shoes are often beveled to increase stability. And that stability is equally important when you roll your foot forward and push off with your toe.

Personally, we recommend walking shoes for serious walkers.

But if you can't find a walking shoe that fits, by all means, try a running shoe. Be sure to go to a store where a knowledgeable salesperson can assist you in selecting a brand and style.

If you're a racewalker, you will have to search until you find a walking shoe that is flexible enough to meet the demands of your sport. Try grabbing the shoe at both ends and bending it. If it doesn't flex easily and you want to go really fast, then shop around for another brand. Some racewalkers prefer running flats, a type of running shoe that is very flexible and has a very thin sole.

pedist. You're worth the expense, and so are your shoes.

Go to a store that carries a wide variety of brands and styles, so you have the best chance of finding the right shoes for your feet. Once you've selected a pair, you can go to other stores to see if you can get the same brand and style for less. Keep your eyes peeled for sales and discounts.

We're not going to tell you our favorite brands and styles, because they may not be the best for *your* feet. But we can tell you a little about some of the major manufacturers.

New Balance is considered to be a leader among manufacturers of footwear. They make lots of sizes and widths to fit all kinds of feet. They also have styles for every foot type.

Easy Spirit shoes are best for rigid or neutral feet, with styles that tend to be a bit softer and more flexible than those of other brands.

Saucony walking shoes are known for their ability to keep people from overpronating. They have a special insert that acts like a soft orthotic, which provides great arch support. (An orthotic is a device that holds your foot in a biomechanically correct position.)

Other big names in the walking-shoe industry include Rykä, Etonic, Natural-Sport, Nike, Reebok, Adidas, Wilson, Brooks, Rockport, and Asics. Some of these brands, such as Nike, are available only in B widths. Other brands are available in a variety of widths, but

---

Shoe-Shopping Strategies

In the market for a new pair of walking shoes? *Caveat emptor* has a new meaning for people with diabetes who are buying shoes. It can be a life- or limb-saving decision.

"Feet are a weak point in anyone with diabetes," says Stephen G. Rosen, MD, chief of endocrinology at Pennsylvania Hospital in Philadelphia. "People with diabetes who take up walking need to buy sturdy, well-constructed shoes."

Follow these shopping guidelines to find the perfect match for your feet.

- Shop at the end of the day, when your feet are largest. As the day goes on, feet tend to swell a little bit. You may actually be a half size larger in the afternoon than in the morning. Footwear that's too small can cause all kinds of problems. Several years ago, a study by the American Podiatric Medical Association revealed that most foot problems among women result from wearing shoes that are too small.

- "When shopping for walking shoes, have your feet properly measured," says John M. Giurini, DPM, president-elect of the American College of Foot and Ankle Surgeons and associate professor in surgery at Harvard Medical School in Boston. "Your feet change over time, so even if you've 'always' worn a size $8\frac{1}{2}$, now you may need a $9\frac{1}{2}$."

- Wear your walking socks. Some styles are really thick, and you may need to go a half-size larger with your shoes to accommodate them.

stores don't bother to stock them. If a store doesn't carry the style that you want in the width that will fit you best, don't hesitate to order a pair. You still get to try them on when they come in. Don't let an overeager salesperson try to persuade you otherwise.

So, wise consumer, go forth with your new shoe knowledge and shop. Once you've gotten your feet into some serious walking shoes, you're ready to begin a serious walking program.

- When you try on shoes, make sure that there's plenty of room—at least a finger's width—beyond the end of your longest toe (usually the big toe). Measure when you're standing up rather than sitting down.

- "You may have to throw vanity out the window," says Dr. Giurini. "Look for a supportive shoe with a rigid heel counter for the best heel and ankle support. Choose a shoe with a thick cushioned sole, either a crepe sole or Vibram, because they provide a little protection and shock absorption. Stay away from thin, leather soles. Look for a soft upper that will give and expand, rather than rigid, patent leather. And if you have any foot problems such as hammertoes, choose shoes to accommodate that."

- Spend some time in the shoes you are trying on. Walk around the store. If you're in a mall, ask if you can take a few laps around the inside corridors. The shoes should feel great. In addition, a skilled shoe salesperson should be able to watch you walk and assess whether the shoes are giving you enough support.

- "Buy tie shoes, as opposed to loafers. They tend to support feet better, so your feet slip and slide around less inside them," says Dr. Giurini. "Also, look for a walking or jogging shoe made from a combination of nylon and leather. They're lightweight and breathe more than all-leather shoes."

- "The American Podiatric Medical Association recommends footwear with the APMA Seal of Acceptance," adds Robert Katz, DPM, a podiatrist in Bradenton, Florida.

CHAPTER 9

GETTING ALL GEARED UP

Besides a good pair of walking shoes, what else might you need to dedicate yourself to a regular walking program? Actually, not much. Of course, you can always find stuff to buy—more gear, more gadgets—and some of it is lots of fun. But if you're a beginning walker, you probably already own most of what you need. And what you don't own you should be able to buy relatively inexpensively.

EXTRA PROTECTION FOR YOUR SOLES

Next to your shoes, your socks are your most important piece of walking gear. A lousy pair of socks can make a great pair of shoes feel absolutely awful. On the other hand, an okay pair of shoes can feel a lot more tolerable when they're worn over a fantastic pair of socks.

The sock market has exploded in the past few decades, beginning with a brand called Thorlo. As far as we know, Thorlo was the first company to realize that because human feet lose their fatty padding as they get older, folks would appreciate a little cushioning in their socks. Thorlo walking socks are thick and luxurious, with extra padding in the ball and heel. You feel as if you're walking on a cloud, provided your walking shoes are big enough to accommodate all that fluff. Otherwise, you just feel cramped.

Like any good athletic sock, Thorlo walking socks are synthetic. They wick away sweat from your feet, dry quickly, and retain their shape, softness, and resiliency. As a rule, socks made from synthetic fabrics are best. A little cotton is okay, but all-cotton socks get soggy, lose their shape and softness, and wear through faster.

These days, Thorlo has lots of company in the walking-sock category. Many stores carry dizzying displays of socks in all brands, colors, sizes, and styles. Some are thick; some are thin. Some support your arch; others pad your bunion. Many footwear manufacturers offer socks bearing the same brand names as their shoes.

Our suggestion is to try a variety of brands and styles until you find one that you really like. Then buy a whole bunch, so you always have a clean pair waiting for you. Few things feel better than slipping on fresh, soft, padded socks first thing in the morning.

Wonder what type of socks a podiatrist wears? "I like synthetic and cotton blended white socks because they will wick away moisture as well as provide good comfort," says Robert Katz, DPM, a podiatrist in Bradenton, Florida. "Socks without seams are best."

When you're going for a long walk—say, more than 4 miles—you may want to carry an extra pair of socks with you. Then if your feet get hot or wet, just change socks. You'll feel totally refreshed and revitalized.

IN CLOTHING, COMFORT BEATS FASHION

Now that you have your feet properly attired, what about the rest of you? Let the temperature outside be your guide when you're deciding what to wear.

For warm-weather walking, you need a pair of comfortable shorts that won't ride up the inside of your legs. We prefer stretch shorts, such as those worn for cycling. On top, a T-shirt is fine. We like the kinds that are cotton-polyester blends. They're softer than 100 percent cotton shirts, and they don't shrink.

Speaking of T-shirts: As you become more involved in walking and attend events or races, you'll get more Ts than you know what to do with. Rather than stuffing them into the back of your closet, you could have some of them made into a beautiful memory quilt.

For cooler weather, sweatpants or stretch pants are great. Choose a fabric that breathes and wicks away sweat, such as Lycra spandex. Make sure that your pants allow for a full range of motion.

Treadmills: The Ultimate Walking Gear

A treadmill might be a worthy addition to your walking program. While you don't want to walk inside all the time, using a treadmill may be the only way for you to exercise with the consistency necessary to achieve the health and fitness benefits you desire.

Treadmills range in price from $130 to $5,000. How much you spend depends on how many functions and features you want. More expensive models usually come loaded with an array of electronic extras, plus they have great stability and durability. They're able to meet the demands of even the most punishing walkers.

We're not going to recommend specific models here because brands and styles change so rapidly. We advise against buying a treadmill that doesn't have a motor. Though these machines tend to be cheaper and much quieter than motorized models, most people who try them just don't like the effort required to start them and keep them going.

The kind of motorized treadmill that will serve you best depends on your age, your fitness level, and your goals. Keep these guidelines in mind when you're shopping around.

- Basic functions and features: good deck stability (the deck is the part of the machine that you walk on), comfortable adjustments for starting and stopping, smooth speed changes, easy-to-use programs, at least one interval-training program to vary your routine, heart rate monitor
- Needs for people age 50 and over: quick and easy manual modes for getting started; gradual and gentle starting, stopping, and pace changes; simple electronics; large, easy-to-read screen displays
- Needs for people under age 50: quick start and program override functions, more variety in programs, customizable programs, wide range of speed and incline changes

For first-timers, walking on a treadmill can take some getting used to. To help you start out smoothly and safely, use this step-by-step approach suggested by Mark Bricklin, former editor-in-chief of *Prevention* magazine and an avid 'miller.

1. Plant your feet on the side rails and grip the handrails. To avoid motor strain, don't step on the belt until the speed reaches about 1 mile per hour.

2. Keep a light grip on the handrails for a while. Once you're comfortable, let your arms swing naturally at your sides.

3. Slowly increase the speed until you're walking at a comfortable pace.

4. After a few minutes, with the incline set flat, increase the speed a tad. Keep swinging those arms.

5. Position yourself so that the control panel is within easy reach. Never let yourself drift backward; some people have been flipped off the back of these machines.

6. Listen to your feet: Are they going *poom, poom, poom*? If so, you're landing flat-footed. Try landing on your heel and rolling your foot forward.

7. Check where your feet are pointing. If they're aiming outward, try to position them so that they're straight ahead. Why walk in two directions at once?

8. If you're in front of a mirror, watch your head. Are you bobbing up and down? If so, your stride is probably too long. Shorten it for a smooth, gliding walk.

9. Make sure you're not leaning forward from the waist. It strains your back.

10. Maintain a pace that leaves you feeling invigorated.

11. If your treadmill has an incline function, use it to add oomph to your workout in short bursts—anywhere from 30 seconds to 3 minutes. When walking becomes laborious or you start losing good form, return to a flat position.

12. When you're ready to stop, ease up your pace and walk slowly for a few minutes. Then step onto the side rails and turn off the treadmill. When you get off, you're going to feel a little dizzy. It's natural. Grab a drink of water and allow yourself a few minutes to regain your "shore legs."

Avoid those that are too tight around the waist. You need to breathe. On top, you may want a long-sleeved T-shirt and a lightweight jacket, depending on the temperature. (If you're heading out in really cold weather, check out the tips in Chapter 13.)

A HEADS-UP FOR GOOD POSTURE

To complete your walking outfit, you'll want to have a hat, a visor, or a pair of sunglasses. It's not just to protect your eyes from the glare of the sun or to save your skin from wrinkles—though those are nice bonuses. When the sun is shining brightly, many people tilt their heads down to avoid a glare directly in their eyes. Walking in that position creates extra strain in the neck and upper back.

What's more, looking down at the ground is more likely to leave you feeling down. When you wear a hat, a visor, or sunglasses, you keep your chin up, literally and figuratively.

One brand of visors is ScrunchVisor, which is made by DesignWear. They have an ultralight, supersoft foam brim that rolls up and can easily fit in a pocket or fanny pack. They come equipped with a Velcro closure, so they can be adjusted to your head size and hairstyle. The visors have sewn-in sweatbands and are completely washable.

DesignWear also makes scrunchable baseball caps. For more information or to place an order, visit www.scrunchwear. com.

THE PERFECT PACK FOR PERAMBULATING

When you're walking, you want to be able to swing your arms freely. For this reason, you really shouldn't carry anything, not even a water bottle or a CD player. But you may have a few items—your house or car keys, money, medication, or tissues— that you want to keep with you. That's when a fanny pack can come in handy.

Hanging loosely around your waist, a fanny pack is wonderful. Some fanny packs are designed to accommodate water bottles. In fact, L. L. Bean makes one that holds two bottles.

When fanny packs first became popular, they were worn behind the body, over the fanny (hence their name). That may be the best placement when you're walking briskly. But if you're shopping or traveling, or anywhere you're feeling

Don't Leave Home without It

For people with diabetes, the most critical piece of their walking gear is their identification.

"It's important for people with diabetes to have identification on them if they're walking," says Kashif Munir, MD, an endocrinologist and medical director of the Joslin Diabetes Center at Baltimore Washington Medical Center in Glen Burnie, Maryland. "Wear a necklace or wristband that tells that you have diabetes and if you are on insulin. That's critical if something happens to you and you're not able to communicate."

the slightest bit unsafe, wear the pack on the front of your body. It's more secure and accessible in that position.

If you're going for a walk and you don't need to carry more than a key and your ID (which you should *always* have with you), you might be able to make do with a wrist wallet. Some styles are made from terry cloth, with Velcro closures that secure around your wrist. These wallets are useful if your workout wear doesn't have any pockets.

KEEPING THE PACE WITH YOUR TIMEPIECE

You may not think of your watch as walking gear. But it can become an indispens-

able part of your workout—and not just for showing you when it's time to turn around and head for home. Using your watch, you can determine your pace— that is, how fast you cover a mile.

If you're walking on a measured course, you can time each mile of your workouts and use that to track improvements in your speed and strength. Plus, as you get to know how it feels to walk at a certain pace—to cover a mile in a certain number of minutes—you'll be able to judge fairly accurately how far you've gone, based on how much time you've spent walking.

If you cover a mile in 20 minutes, you're moving at a pace of 3 miles per hour. That's a comfortable speed for any-

Low-Tech Pulse-Checking

Keeping tabs on your heart rate is easy, and you don't need a heart monitor to do it. A watch with a second hand works just as well.

First, you need to find your pulse. Place the index and middle fingers of one hand against the carotid artery, located at the front of your neck. Press just hard enough that you can pick up the sensation of your pulse. Count the beats for 10 seconds, timing yourself with your watch.

If you've been walking really fast, keep moving slowly while you check your pulse. Stopping suddenly can cause your heart to skip beats, which can be very distressing, especially if you have a heart problem.

Once you've counted the number of beats, compare it with the 10-second heart-rate range for your age group. In the chart below, all of the ranges have been calculated to reflect 70 to 80 percent of your maximum heart rate. Memorize your 10-second range, so you'll know what to aim for when you're working out.

Keep in mind that 70 to 80 percent of your maximum heart rate is a high-intensity workout. If you're within your target range, that's great, but you can still get a good workout at a lower heart rate.

As a general rule, you should be able to carry on a conversation while you're walking, even if you have to huff and puff a little to do it. If you're breathless, you're going too fast for your fitness level.

AGE	EXERCISING HEART-RATE RANGE	RANGE FOR A 10-SECOND COUNT
35–39	130–148	22–25
40–44	126–144	21–24
45–49	123–140	21–23
50–54	119–136	20–23
55–59	116–132	19–22
60–64	112–128	19–21
65+	109–124	18–21

one who is in good health and exercises a couple of times a week.

If you walk a mile in 15 minutes, you have a pace of 4 miles per hour. That's considered brisk. Most people need to work up to a 15-minute mile. Going that fast feels somewhat challenging and exhilarating. You're breathing noticeably faster, but you're most likely able to carry on a conversation. You just can't sing an aria.

If you cover a mile in 12 minutes, you're cruising at a pace of 5 miles per hour. At that speed, walking starts to become inefficient from a biomechanical standpoint. It just feels very hard. In fact, running would be easier if you can tolerate the pounding on your joints. If not, you may have to use some sort of special technique, such as racewalking, to keep up.

As you might imagine, increasing your pace—going from a 20-minute mile to a 15-minute mile, for example—takes effort. If you slack off, you'll have to work to regain your strength and endurance. At those speeds, you will make great strides in fitness. But going fast isn't necessary if your main goal is better health. Many people do between 15- and 20-minute miles, and they're very comfortable at that pace.

But who knows? You may decide to train for a 5-K and start pushing yourself harder . . . for the fun of it!

THE PROS AND CONS OF PEDOMETERS

Some walkers put pedometers in the "frill gear" category. But others like these gadgets. They work by counting the number of steps you take, ticking off a step every time you move your leg. Then they multiply that figure by the length of your stride to get your mileage.

The problem is, your stride changes when you encounter hills. You may lengthen your stride going uphill and shorten it on the way down. But a pedometer can't make that same adjustment. So if a group of people went walking, with everyone wearing the same type of pedometer, they may end up with different mileages for the same route. Hopefully, each pedometer would be within 1/4 mile of the correct mileage.

If you buy a pedometer, consider one that is totally mechanical. That way, you don't have to worry about replacing batteries. Besides, mechanical models are easy to read, and they don't have as many buttons and functions.

With any pedometer, the tricky part is setting it to your stride length. Here's the best way.

1. Mark off a level 20-foot-long path.
2. Walk that distance, counting the number of steps you take. Give yourself room for a walking start, so you're using a relaxed, normal gait by the time you reach the marked-off path.
3. Divide the distance (20 feet) by the number of steps to determine your stride length. For example, if you took 10 steps, divide 20 by 10 for a stride length of 2 feet.
4. Repeat this process three times. Then use those results to calculate an average stride length.
5. Set your pedometer to that stride length.

FOR THE HARDWORKING HEART . . .

With all the technological advances now taking place, the day will come when you can buy endless varieties of devices to track not only your pace but also your heart rate and your respiration rate. Already, you can wear a continuous glucose monitoring system to check your blood sugar level while you walk. But unless you have a specific health problem that requires you to constantly monitor your vital signs, such features certainly aren't necessary.

These high-tech gadgets might be helpful for someone who is recovering from a heart attack or who has a heart problem, for example. But if you're a beginning walker without heart problems, simple pulse-taking techniques should provide all the monitoring you need.

That said, if you'd like to bump your fitness level up a notch or two, or if you want to burn more calories while you walk, a heart monitor can be a great tool to help you along. You can set the monitor to beep as soon as you drop below your target heart rate range, alerting you to pick up your pace. Likewise, if you exceed the high end of your range, the monitor will beep to let you know that you're pushing too hard, which only tires you out more quickly.

Some heart monitors fit on a finger; others are strapped around the chest or fitted into a special bra. Basic models begin at about $50 and are available online and in sporting goods/fitness equipment stores, health clubs, and some department stores.

Chapter 10

FINDING THE BEST PLACE
AND THE BEST TIME

We've already addressed the "what" of walking: what you need and what you don't. So let's move on to the next most-pressing questions: when and where?

The simple answer is, you can go for a walk anytime you want, anywhere you want. That's what makes walking such a great activity: its convenience.

But if you're just starting a walking program and you're trying to make it a habit, then you need to do a little more planning. You can't rely on a spur-of-the-moment urge to take a walk, unless you naturally get those urges every day.

LOCATION MAKES A DIFFERENCE

The best place to do your walking is the one that you find most attractive *and* most convenient. These two qualities are inseparable.

You may know a wonderful trail through a beautiful park across town. But if driving there takes you 20 minutes, are you willing to make that trip every day or several days a week? Or perhaps there's a path close to your workplace, but it's littered with trash and so close to traffic that you'd be inhaling exhaust fumes instead of fresh air. Do you really want to give up your afternoon coffee and doughnut for that—even if walking on your break time would be a healthier and more reliable pick-me-up than snacking?

If you can walk out your front door to a sidewalk that takes you safely around your neighborhood, that's great. But if you live in an area with no sidewalks and cars going around blind curves at 50 miles an hour, you'll have to get creative.

If you can't walk close to home, or you simply prefer not to, consider these venues instead.

Municipal parks: You may find that the best place to walk is in a nearby municipal park. These usually provide bathroom facilities and water fountains. And many have mileage markers, so you can monitor your distance and check your pace. Just try to avoid parks where walkers and cyclists share the same paths. Mixed-use trails can be very hazardous, especially for walkers who are talking or wearing headphones and don't hear cyclists speeding up behind them. A collision can cause serious injury or worse to everyone involved.

County and state parks: Check out other local natural resources, too. Some may be closer than you think. For example, many county- and state-run parks have great walking and hiking trails. Call your local parks and recreation department to request maps. Also find out whether the trails are considered safe for solitary walkers or you're better off with a partner. In general, if lots of people use the trails, there's safety in numbers. If a park is all but deserted, you might want to think twice before going there on your own.

Tracks: High school and college tracks are great when you want to work on your walking technique, when you are trying to improve your speed, or when you just want to get in your miles and go home. If you're on a track for the first time, you may want to see how long it takes you to do a mile—that's four laps—at a comfortable pace. Also, check whether your local YMCA or health club has an indoor track, which is ideal for days when you don't want to walk outside. If the track is sloped, be sure to change directions often to avoid straining one leg.

Malls: More walkers are taking advantage of the temperature-controlled, traffic-free environment at their local malls. Often these people are "regulars" who are looking for a little camaraderie as well as exercise. As a bonus, they have ready access to bathrooms, water fountains, telephones, and even food. Many malls open their doors early to walkers who want to get in their workouts before the stores open and shoppers arrive. To find out whether your local mall has such a policy, just call the administrative office.

CHANGE COURSE? IT'S YOUR CHOICE

Should you walk the same route every day, or should you switch routes from one day to the next? That's really up to you. Do what keeps you interested. It makes sticking with a walking program a whole lot easier.

Some walkers prefer to stay on one route. They like to watch the changes from day to day and from season to season. Or they look forward to interacting with certain people or animals that they meet along the way. Or they appreciate the familiarity of the route because they can relax and let their minds drift, perhaps to mull over problems and come up with solutions.

Other walkers need to change routes to keep themselves stimulated and entertained. They look for new, convenient walking paths. They like the excitement of wondering what's around the next bend. They get a kick out of discovering new paths. So think about your own likes and interests, then spend some time finding routes that suit your personal preferences.

TIMING IS EVERYTHING

Once you've settled on where you want to walk, you need to decide when.

Diabetes will likely factor into that choice. "If you have diabetes, the best time to walk is after you eat," says Stephen G. Rosen, MD, chief of endocrinology at Pennsylvania Hospital in Philadelphia.

Quick Tip

If you walk in a multistory mall, you can use the open stairwells to boost your calorie burn and build stronger leg muscles. For an even more intense workout, climb the escalators before they're turned on in the morning. But use caution: Escalator steps can be deeper than standard steps, and the metal treads can catch sneakers. Be sure to wear walking or running shoes.

The Mall Calls

For a safe, comfortable workout, no place beats the local mall. Like walking outdoors, walking at the mall is free. What's more, it burns extra calories.

In a study of 60 women and men who were timed with a stopwatch when they walked, researchers found that the women naturally walked faster in a mall than on a track. And the faster you move, the more calories you burn.

"Where you walk makes a difference," says study author Richard S. Cimbalo, PhD, professor of psychology at Daemen College in Amherst, New York. "Something about the mall—possibly that it's a familiar and safe place—may help women get a better workout."

But that's not the only advantage to walking in a mall. Here are some other reasons why you may want to take your exercise indoors.

You're too hot. When the temperature rises above 75°F, your heart has to work twice as hard to deliver blood not only to the muscles you're using, but also to your skin to keep it cool. "Anybody who's at risk for heart disease shouldn't be exercising outdoors in those conditions," advises Bryant Stamford, PhD, director of the Health Promotion Center at the University of Louisville in Kentucky.

"That's when you are less likely to have a low blood sugar reaction."

People with a lot of swelling may benefit by walking in the morning because their swelling will increase as the day progresses, says Robert Katz, DPM, a podiatrist in Bradenton, Florida. Keep in mind, though, that if you walk in the morning, you need to stretch well because the risk for injury is greater in the morning due to increased strain on tight muscles.

Another factor to consider is that most experts will tell you that if you want to be consistent, your best bet is to walk in the morning. By getting it out of the way early, there's less chance of your workout being sidelined by other obligations that arise over the course of a day.

If this works for you, fantastic. Many

You're too cold. Cold presents its own problems, which may be complicated by icy or snowy sidewalks. Often, it's safer to drive than it is to walk. So drive yourself to the mall and walk there.

You're sneezing. In most malls, the air is filtered as well as cool and dry. So if you have allergies, you won't be bothered by pollen or dust as you would outdoors.

You like company. Many malls sponsor organized walking programs, which may include group walks, special incentives, and even speakers and health fairs. To find out whether your local mall has such a program, call or stop by the administrative office.

You have trouble staying motivated. Mall walkers are a fiercely devoted bunch. "If you stop showing up, they're going to call to find out where you are," says Sara Donovan, founder of WalkSport America, a Minnesota company that manages mall-walking programs such as the one at Mall of America.

You want security. A mall offers a smooth, even walking surface that's well-lit and well-populated. You can feel safe there. That's one of the big reasons why mall walking has become so popular, even in areas where the climate is mild.

You're short on cash. Walking in a mall is a lot less expensive than joining a health club or buying a treadmill.

people find that an early-morning walk makes a great start to a productive day. By the time they finish their workouts, they feel relaxed and energized. Plus, if you get out the door early enough, you'll beat the early-morning commuters. That means there's less traffic and less car exhaust to deal with.

If you're not a morning person, don't force yourself to become one. You need to find a time to walk that suits your schedule and your lifestyle. As with choosing the right place, choosing the right time can make committing to a walking program much easier.

For you, lunch-time may be the perfect time to walk, especially if you work outside your home and you have young children or other responsibilities that keep you from getting out of the house early in the morning or after dinner. For working parents, a lunch-hour workout can seem like a mini-vacation. It provides a great opportunity for you to de-stress.

If you and your spouse like to exercise together, you may prefer to take after-

Road Hazards

From Dodges to dogs, the road can be a dangerous place for walkers. But that's no excuse to stay inside on the couch. Here's a troubleshooter's guide to the most common walking hazards.

SUV versus You

Rule #1: Walk against the flow of traffic, on the left-hand side of the road, so you'll see cars coming at you.

Rule #2: Never assume a driver sees you. When you need to cross, make eye contact with the driver and wait for him to wave you on.

Rule #3: When walking at night, wear a flashing light and shoes and clothes bearing reflective stripes. According to AAA tests, drivers can clearly see reflective strips from 700 feet, more than twice the length of a football field. In comparison, they can see fluorescent clothing only from 100 feet.

Bad Dog

If a dog gives chase, the best thing to do is stop walking, make a quarter turn, and walk away, says Dennis Fetko, PhD, an animal behaviorist and trainer. "By changing your body orientation slightly, you let the dog know, in a nonthreatening way, that you know he's there and that you're prepared to defend yourself if he attacks." You want to keep moving because the farther you get from his territory, the less likely he is to follow you. Never turn and stare down the dog; he'll think you want to attack him.

dinner walks. They're a wonderful opportunity for the two of you to spend time together and to discuss the day's events away from the dishes, the telephone, and the TV. Many couples describe walking as the balm that soothed a raw nerve in their

---

For extra protection, carry a bottle of Direct Stop (around $10). When sprayed in a dog's face, it overwhelms him with the scent of citronella, disorienting him for 30 seconds or so.

A Pain in the Knee

Switch to the other side of the road. Changing the angle of the road surface (most streets slope slightly) will relieve pressure on your knee. If that doesn't help, move to a more yielding surface, such as a dirt path, which isn't as hard as asphalt, says Rick Braver, DPM, a sports podiatrist in New Jersey.

Still feeling pain? Stop walking and sit down with your legs straight in front of you. Tighten your quads for 2 seconds, then release. Repeat 5 times. "This helps squeeze out excess fluid around the kneecap, which may be causing pain, and releases synovial fluid, which lubricates the knee to reduce pain," says Dr. Braver. If the knee still hurts, walk home. Consider seeing your doctor.

Lightning

If you can't get inside a building, head for a car or other fully enclosed structure. Partially open structures are no good, says Mary Ann Cooper, MD, head of the Lightning Injury Research Program at the University of Illinois at Chicago. Avoid open spots, because you could be the tallest thing in the area. Stay away from water and tall objects, including trees.

To figure out how close lightning is (in miles), count the number of seconds between the lightning and the thunder, then divide by 5. Right before lightning strikes, you may feel your hair stand on end or hear some staticky noise.

relationships. Just plan on going at a leisurely pace. When you walk after a meal, your body is putting all of its energy into digesting food. If you walk too fast, you may end up with cramps or indigestion.

Depending on your schedule, you may have to do your walking just before bedtime. Keep in mind that walking at night isn't for everyone. While some say that it's the perfect nightcap, others find it too stimulating. Safety is an issue, too. Experiment to find out whether it's right for you.

GET IT IN WRITING

Choosing a time to walk is relatively easy. Sticking with it may be more of a challenge. These days, so many of us have such tightly packed schedules that we wonder how we can possibly add even one more item to our "to do" lists.

If you keep an appointment book, make walking one of your appointments. Or write a note on each day of your wall calendar: "Walk at 7:30 a.m." That way, you have a constant reminder of your commitment to exercising and getting fit.

And each time you go walking, don't forget to mark it off in your appointment book or on your calendar. It shows not only that you scheduled your workout but also that you actually followed through. If you're a more spontaneous type who squeezes in walks whenever you can, then write them down after the fact. For example, you could keep track of your workouts in your daily planner. And if you notice that you're skipping days, then you might want to start scheduling your walks. That will help you remember how important consistency is and how much better you feel when you exercise regularly.

CHAPTER 11

PAIRING UP
FOR EXERCISE SUCCESS

To reap all of the physical and mental benefits of walking, you need to do it every day—or almost every day—for the rest of your life. That's a tall order, even for a dedicated walker. Some days you'll be short on time, energy, or motivation, and you'll need a little extra nudge to put on your walking shoes. Other days you'll be short on all three, and you'll need a big push. But chances are, once you're out walking, you'll feel great.

Even if you enjoy the solitude of your walks, sometimes a buddy may help to get you going. Teaming up with a partner keeps your motivation from sliding and your walking program on track, even when you're convinced that you have other "more important" things to do. On days when it's too cold, warm, or wet outside and you're looking for an excuse not to walk, a partner can motivate you to do it anyway.

Of course, you can undertake a walking program on your own if you want. But studies show that few people stick with a fitness routine of any kind unless they have a partner. We humans need social support. Even when we join walking groups, we usually do it with someone else.

If you have a chronic medical condition such as diabetes, you have an even more compelling reason to walk with a buddy. "For someone with diabetes, exercising with a partner is a safety issue," says Stephen G. Rosen, MD, chief of endocrinology at Pennsylvania Hospital in Philadelphia. "The partner needs to know you have diabetes and what to do in case of an emergency."

Anyone can become your walking partner: a family member, a friend, a co-worker, or a neighbor. Be open to whomever happens to come your way. You may not find one person who's willing to walk with you every day. But you can likely recruit two or three people, each of whom can keep you company at various times throughout the week.

To maintain your motivation, you and your most frequent walking partner should share the same agenda. Maybe both of you want to lose weight, improve your fitness level, or work off stress. Or maybe you enjoy bird-watching or window-shopping while you walk. Whatever your mutual goals or pleasures, they'll keep the two of you coming together for regular, consistent workouts.

STEPPING OUT WITH YOUR SPOUSE

When you're looking for a walking partner, you may want to start your search close to home. That way, each time you exercise, you have an opportunity to strengthen the relationships that are most important in your life, those that contribute to your sense of happiness and well-being.

If you're married, you may want to ask your spouse to walk with you. Some marriage counselors believe that walking together can improve the way that you and your significant other relate to one another. So you not only add miles to your exercise log, you also bring harmony into your home. You could call it sweat bonding.

How can walking strengthen marital ties? For one thing, it removes you from all the duties and distractions that take the fun and romance out of a marriage—things like paying bills and doing household chores. For another, when done outside in the sunshine, it raises levels of a feel-good brain chemical called serotonin. Serotonin helps adjust your frame of mind, so you're better able to address any issues that you and your spouse might want to discuss.

Walking also stimulates the release of the mood-boosting compounds known as endorphins. You feel more optimistic, more upbeat—and if you're with your spouse, you may associate the good feelings with him or her. You may see the other person in a more positive light, which can help smooth over any anger or disenchantment with your relationship.

In fact, many couples say that they

have an easier time communicating with each other when they're walking. They're more comfortable opening up to their partners because they're side by side rather than face-to-face. And because walking can release tension, they're more likely to feel calm while discussing sensitive or divisive issues.

In Step with Mary Nagle

Getting Fit on the Buddy System

Long before walking became America's favorite fitness activity, Mary Nagle was pounding the highways and byways around her country home. She tries to walk at least once every day.

What keeps the Zionsville, Pennsylvania, resident on such an ambitious schedule? "I always find a partner," she says. "My friends in the neighborhood are just as enthusiastic about walking, and we call each other the night before to set up a time and place to meet."

Mary first took up walking as a way to control her weight. But among her female companions, she soon found herself using her workouts to blow off steam. "Sometimes I just want to vent, and my women friends understand that," she says. "I'd never feel comfortable letting go like that in front of their husbands."

Over time, Mary's walks have become what she describes as a positive addiction. "If I can't go walking, for whatever reason, I find myself getting moody and anxious," she explains.

These days, Mary meets at least one of her walking buddies at 7:30 every morning—rain, sleet, or snow. "Actually, I love walking in the snow because I can always dress warm for cold weather," she says. "Staying cool is a bit more difficult, but I've figured out a way to do it. When the weather gets hot, I wrap ice cubes in paper towels and tuck them inside my bra."

For Mary, having a walking partner is key to sticking with her walking program. "I feel bored or lazy when I'm alone," she says. "But when I make a commitment and I know that Carolyn, Sarita, Ann, or Peggy is waiting for me, I'm always there."

If you and your spouse use your walks to reminisce about your relationship, the two of you may remember what brought you together in the first place. That's important, because as one marriage counselor points out, spouses today tend to think of themselves as married "singles" rather than as married couples. By walking together, you and your spouse may see each other as "we," not as "you and me."

CONNECTING WITH KIDS

If you and your spouse can't always walk together, ask your child or grandchild to join you instead. Kids can be great walking partners, provided you choose a destination that's of interest to them.

Don't just suggest going for a walk; there's a good chance that you'll be ignored. Instead, offer it as a trip to a video arcade, an ice-cream parlor, a school playground, or a park. Most youngsters will gladly go the distance if the end goal seems enticing enough. But most important, you'll have lots of fun—and get plenty of exercise—en route.

If you're walking with very young children, remember this: You're the one with the ability to adapt. Slow down to match the child's pace. Walk too fast or too far, and the child may not want to go with you again.

And don't view your stroll as an opportunity to lecture to a captive audience. Just smile and relax. Let the kids do the talking, and enjoy their company.

WALKING ON THE JOB

Outside your family, you may be able to find a walking partner or two among your co-workers. The workplace can be fertile ground for walkers. Everyone gets breaks, and using that time to go walking can do more to de-stress and reenergize you than coffee and a doughnut.

Try to block out at least part of your lunch hour for walking, too. You definitely don't want to skip your lunch completely, but save 10 to 15 minutes for a walk. It can be a great stress reliever. (Ideally, you should eat after your walk, so you don't tax your digestive system. If you opt to eat first, keep your pace leisurely to avoid cramps and indigestion.)

Keep an extra pair of walking shoes and socks at your desk, so you can be ready at a moment's notice. For really brisk walking on warm days, you may want to change into workout clothes. But on cool days, just slip on your shoes and socks.

Try to choose a walking partner who is a good match for you in terms of fitness level, pace, and stamina. You may want to have several partners—one who likes to stroll when you don't want to work up a sweat, another who's up for a half hour of hill walking when you want more of a workout. Just don't push yourself to keep up with someone who walks a lot faster than you. It isn't worth the risk of injury. If you're gasping for breath while your partner conducts most of the conversation, you need to slow down.

Walking with co-workers gives you an opportunity to get to know each other away from on-the-job pressures. You improve your rapport with fellow employees—and get a better-toned body to boot.

PARTNER WITH A POOCH

When you're in the market for a walking partner, don't overlook the four-legged variety. Fido, of course, isn't going to call 911 for you in the case of a medical emergency. So a dog isn't a substitute for a walking buddy. But a dog certainly can add motivation and fun to your walks.

Walking with a dog isn't for everyone, and we certainly don't advise adopting a dog just for your walking program. Pet ownership is a big responsibility. But a pooch can be a most devoted and reliable walking partner.

The great thing about dogs is that they *always* want to go for a walk. And they make wonderful company: If you want to talk, dogs will listen without complaint; if you prefer to walk in silence, they won't feel slighted.

Some dogs need obedience training to prepare them for a walking partnership. But most are natural, able partners right from the start. If you have a dog that hasn't been exercising regularly, get him checked out by a veterinarian first. Ask the vet to recommend a training program to ease your dog into exercise.

If you don't currently have a dog and would like to adopt one, a veterinarian or kennel club can help you find the breed that best suits your lifestyle. Ideally, you want a dog that's friendly to other people and to other dogs, one that is strong and can tolerate the temperatures where you live.

If you just want a walking partner, not necessarily a full-time companion, ask friends and neighbors if you can "borrow" their dogs. Or contact your local animal shelter; often they're in need of volunteer dog-walkers.

Part III

WALK IN
ANY WEATHER

Chapter 12

KEEP YOUR COOL IN THE HEAT

When it's so hot outside you start to sweat just thinking about going out for a walk, don't do it. But that's no excuse to settle in on the couch with Oprah and Gayle. When the heat is stifling, your best bet is to move your workout inside to an indoor track or a treadmill. Or you can do your walking in a pool, if you have access to one.

Heat can be dangerous. Some days it may be hotter than you think. No matter what the reading on the thermometer, the temperature can feel even higher to your body. And that can have serious consequences if you're not careful. Because heat can increase metabolism and affect blood sugar, it can be a big issue for people with diabetes.

WHEN IS HOT TOO HOT?

Sometimes it's tough to tell when a nice, warm day is actually too hot for safe outdoor exercise. You've no doubt learned from experience that high humidity makes a high air temperature feel even more uncomfortable. The combination of humidity and air temperature is known as *apparent temperature*. And as it rises, so does your risk of heat exhaustion or heatstroke, which can be life-threatening.

Heat-related health problems most often affect those who are older and those who have chronic medical conditions. (As spring turns to summer, it's a good idea to have a chat with your doctor about whether you should exercise indoors or forgo your workout altogether.) Young children are also vulnerable. But even the fittest among us can fall victim to the heat if we overexert ourselves or become dehydrated.

So when the mercury is rising, use "Your Hot-Weather Workout Guide" on page 88 to determine whether to do your walking outside or inside (preferably in the air-conditioning). Once you find the day's apparent temperature, check it against the recommendations below.

• 90°F and below: Head for the great outdoors.
• 91° to 104°F: Proceed with caution.
• 105° to 129°F: Consider indoor options unless you're acclimated to these conditions.
• 130°F and above: Stay indoors.

WAYS TO STAY COMFORTABLE

If you decide that the conditions outside are suitable for walking, you still want to make sure that you're prepared to handle the heat. Here are some great tips from veteran walkers who've weathered workouts on hot summer days.

Be an early bird or a night owl. "It's important for people with diabetes to avoid exercising during the peak heat of day and walk early in the morning or later in the evening," says Michael See, MS, registered clinical exercise physiologist at the Joslin Diabetes Center in Boston. "This is especially important for people taking insulin. Walk during the cooler times of day."

Take a glance at the sky before setting out, too. Is it cloudy or glaring sunlight? Direct sun can make the temperature feel up to 15°F higher than it really is.

Drink plenty of water. "Especially in hot weather, it's important to prevent dehydration," says Kashif Munir, MD, an endocrinologist and medical director of the Joslin Diabetes Center at Baltimore Washington Medical Center in Glen Burnie, Maryland.

"Blood sugar levels can rise dramatically in response to dehydration," adds Stephen G. Rosen, MD, chief of endocrinology at Pennsylvania Hospital in Philadelphia. "People with diabetes need to be

A Cool Place for Walking

When the temperature is rising, consider moving your walk to the nearest pool. You'll cool off, and you'll double your workout efficiency to boot.

Exercising in water provides 12 times more resistance than exercising in air. It works both halves of opposing muscle groups—for instance, the muscles on the front and back of your thighs. It conditions major and minor muscle groups and enhances your flexibility. And water's soothing, massaging qualities minimize the soreness that may occur when you exercise harder or longer.

Walking in water is easy. Just hop in the pool and start moving. You can work at any depth you're comfortable in, but the deeper the water, the more it will support your weight and massage your body.

Of course, if you can't touch the bottom of the pool with your feet, you're not walking, you're treading water. That's okay. Treading water is a great workout, too.

very careful when it's hot outside. Make sure you're well hydrated; drink regularly before, during, and after exercising. Also check your blood sugar regularly."

Keep a half-full water bottle in the freezer and top it off just before you head out. Take sips regularly while you're walking. Six to 8 ounces of water for every 15 minutes of walking should be enough. As an extra precaution against dehydration, weigh yourself before your walk and again afterward. If you've dropped a pound or two, drink up.

You've lost fluid that is important to your body's cooling system.

Switch to cooler footwear. For warm-weather workouts, you need light-weight, ventilated walking shoes and socks that wick away sweat. People with diabetes should have two pairs of walking shoes. Alternate between them every day so that each pair has a chance to dry out completely between uses. This helps you avoid blisters, fungi, and stinky feet.

Dress lightly. The more skin that's

Your Hot-Weather Workout Guide

To determine the apparent temperature on any given day, find the environmental temperature (that is, the temperature of the outside air) at the top of the chart and the relative humidity on the left-hand side. Then locate the number where the respective column and row meet. That's the apparent temperature.

ENVIRONMENTAL TEMPERATURE (IN FAHRENHEIT)

RELATIVE HUMIDITY	75°	80°	85°	90°	95°	100°	105°	110°
0%	69	73	78	83	87	91	95	99
10%	70	75	80	85	90	95	100	105
20%	72	77	82	87	93	99	105	112
30%	73	78	84	90	96	104	113	123
40%	74	79	86	93	101	110	123	137
50%	75	81	88	96	107	120	135	150
60%	76	82	90	100	114	132	149	
70%	77	85	93	106	124	144		
80%	78	86	97	113	136			
90%	79	88	102	122				
100%	80	91	108					

APPARENT TEMPERATURE (IN FAHRENHEIT)

exposed, the better sweat can evaporate, and that helps keep you cool. Of course, remember to wear sunscreen. Apply it underneath your shirt also because the garment may not block the sun's harmful ultraviolet rays. If it's really hot, or if you don't like wearing tank tops, mist your shirt with a water bottle. The dampness acts like air-conditioning when you're out walking.

Apply some friction protection. Reduce friction in areas where skin rubs against skin—between your toes, between your thighs, and under your arms—with a little petroleum jelly. Or use Runner's Lube, a nonstaining cream made from lanolin, zinc oxide, and benzocaine that prevents itching and soreness. It's sold in many sporting goods stores.

Friction between the toes is a big problem in hot weather for people with diabetes because friction invites blisters. "Absorptive powders such as Zeasorb can be very helpful to reduce the inter-digital friction," says Robert Katz, DPM, a podiatrist in Bradenton, Florida.

Wear a hat rather than a visor. A visor protects your face, but your head can still get hot. Choose a hat that's made from a breathable fabric, such as cotton or a cotton-synthetic blend. If you can, soak it in cool water before putting it on.

Listen to your body. Your body will tell you when you can push yourself and when you need to coast. If you develop a headache or become dizzy or weak, stop exercising and head for a cool place. Drink plenty of cool fluids while you're resting.

Check your feet. "People with diabetes need to be extra careful of their feet when walking in hot weather," says John M. Giurini, DPM, president-elect of the American College of Foot and Ankle Surgeons and associate professor in surgery at Harvard Medical School in Boston. "If your feet perspire, when you get home, get out of those shoes and socks, wash your feet, dry them well, and check them carefully.

"One thing to watch out for is athlete's foot," he continues. "Signs of it are peeling, cracking, scaling between toes, and itching. You can try to medicate it at home with over-the-counter products, but if it persists for longer than 4 or 5 days, have it looked at by a physician. You might have developed a secondary bacterial infection, which is a more serious condition."

Sport Drinks: Better Than Water?

You know that you need to increase your fluid intake when you exercise, especially in the heat. But you just can't get yourself to take more than a few gulps of water. Why not try a sports drink?

People with diabetes need to be cautious. It's true that if something tastes good, you're bound to consume more of it. And sports drinks contain a small amount of sodium, which makes you want to sip even more. (If you're on a sodium-restricted diet, get your doctor's advice. You may have to limit your sodium intake from other foods and beverages.)

Sports drinks have other benefits besides tasting good. They supply less than half the calories of fruit juices. They're absorbed quickly into the bloodstream, so you can exercise longer and avoid postworkout fatigue. And they're easier on your stomach than beverages with higher concentrations of carbohydrates.

However, the challenge for people with diabetes is that exercise can already increase your blood sugar. Drinking a sports drink is going to raise your level even higher. That's why it's important to check your blood sugar level before and after exercise. If you're exercising for more than a half hour, check your level every half hour during exercise as well. Knowing your blood sugar level, you can decide if a sports drink is a good idea or not.

"People respond differently to exercise," says Kashif Munir, MD, an endocrinologist and medical director of the Joslin Diabetes Center at Baltimore Washington Medical Center in Glen Burnie, Maryland. "If your blood sugar level drops during exercise, a sports drink could provide some needed carbohydrates. However, if your blood sugar level rises during exercise, you wouldn't want to drink a sports drink. Have plain water instead."

CHAPTER 13

WINTERIZE YOUR WALKING PROGRAM

For most people, exercising outdoors may be safer in cooler weather than on hot, humid days. Your body temperature rises as you walk, so when it's sultry outside, you're getting a double dose of heat. When it turns cold, on the other hand, you can regulate your internal temperature more easily. If you get too hot while you're working out, just slow your pace, open your jacket, or take off your hat or gloves. You'll solve the problem instantly.

TAKE CARE WHEN THE TEMP DROPS

Even on chilly days, some of us need to take extra precautions before venturing out to exercise.

Cold-weather workouts can be risky for people with diabetes. Because walking in the cold burns more calories to increase warmth, it steps up the body's demands for blood sugar (glucose). While this is a plus for most folks, it can cause those with diabetes to become hypoglycemic. If you have diabetes, ask your doctor for advice on managing your medications or your food intake to regulate your blood sugar level while you exercise.

You also need to be concerned about developing frostbite, because people with diabetes tend to have poor circulation in their extremities. Warm gloves and a hat are essential. Slip on a pair of wool blend socks to keep your feet warm.

If you experience loss of feeling in your feet or fingers while you're walking, head indoors as soon as you can and check whether your skin looks blue. This condition, called cyanosis, is the first sign of frostbite. You need to see your doctor immediately.

"In cold weather, a person with diabetes should wear a more protective shoe such as a hiking boot instead of a tennis shoe," says Robert Katz, DPM, a podiatrist in Bradenton, Florida. "It is in this weather that the diabetic patient needs to be very careful of the potential for creating a blister or ulceration."

Even though you might not get thirsty in the cold like you would in hot weather, it's still important to stay hydrated. "Even in cold weather you can lose water," says Kashif Munir, MD, an endocrinologist and medical director of the Joslin Diabetes Center at Baltimore Washington Medical Center in Glen Burnie, Maryland. Dehydration is especially dangerous for people with diabetes because it can increase blood sugar levels.

If you have any kind of heart problem, you should consult your doctor before working out in the cold. As the air temperature drops, your body responds by

Get Snow-Tire Traction for Your Shoes

Slippery sidewalks keep many people indoors during the winter months. But you can venture outside safely, provided you have the right equipment.

Stabilicers are detachable soles that can make you so sure-footed you'd feel safe walking across a river of ice. Built like sandals with Velcro straps, they slide over your walking shoes quite easily. The top of the sole grips your shoe, while the bottom, which is imbedded with steel cleats, digs into ice and hard snow. They're perfect for winter walking or any slippery situation.

Stabilicers sell for about $50 a pair. You can find online stores that carry them at www.32north.com, or you can buy them in sporting goods stores as well as through mail-order catalogs.

constricting blood vessels, a process that pulls blood toward the trunk to feed your internal organs. When this happens, exercising puts extra strain on your heart as it tries to pump blood to your extremities.

Walking can relieve some of this strain by dilating blood vessels in your legs. The trick is to warm up slowly, to allow your body to adjust to the coldness. If you don't warm up when it's freezing outside, you could set yourself up for angina (severe chest pain) or a heart attack. That's why people have heart attacks when shoveling snow.

When you warm up, do it indoors, before exposing your body to the cold air. This reduces the strain on your heart, because your blood vessels become dilated. You'll feel better about going outside, too, because you'll be warm already.

Frigid temperatures don't mix well with asthma either. If you have this respiratory condition, you already know that inhaling cold air can trigger an attack. (In fact, some people experience asthma-related breathing problems *only* when they work out in cold weather.) Wearing a mask or scarf over your nose

and mouth can help prevent an attack by warming up the air before it reaches your bronchial tubes. That way, the tubes are less likely to go into spasm. If covering your nose and mouth doesn't help, consult your doctor for advice on adjusting your medication for cold-weather workouts.

In fact, if you have any chronic health problem, you may want to check with your doctor before you exercise in the cold. You'll be told what precautions to take, if any. Or you may be advised to do your walking indoors.

LAYERS KEEP OUT THE COLD

If you are heading outdoors, you need to dress for the chilly temperatures. Twenty years ago, that would have meant donning flannel underwear, a wool sweater, wool pants, a heavy wool coat, and thick wool socks. You'd be so bundled up that you could barely move.

These days, when you dress for wintry conditions, less is more. Thanks to an array of high-tech textiles, you can be warm and dry and still have freedom of movement. New fabrics insulate, block the wind, and wick away moisture without bulk or heaviness.

Still, dressing in layers is your best bet. That way, you can adjust your attire as you go, according to the weather and your level of activity. For the innermost layer (the one closest to your skin), choose light garments made from a synthetic fabric such as polypropylene, which wicks away perspiration from your body. That should be topped off with an insulating layer—a sweater, a sweatshirt, or a fleece pullover—for warmth. For the outermost layer, or shell, you want a garment that protects you from wind and rain. The fabric should be waterproof, as opposed to water-resistant (which is designed to keep you dry in a light mist). It should also be breathable—meaning that it allows water vapor to escape without actually letting water in.

The new synthetic fabrics do a better job of keeping you warm and dry than either wool or cotton. When you're shopping for cold-weather walking wear, read clothing labels and try on a variety of garments to get a sense of what's out there. You'll be amazed at how comfortable you can be, even at extremely cold temperatures.

FOOTWEAR FOR NASTY WEATHER

To prepare your feet for winter walking, often all you need is a pair of walking shoes and a thick pair of socks. Then as you warm up, your feet warm up, too. Just make sure that your shoes can accommodate your socks, or your feet will get cold from lack of circulation.

For keeping your feet toasty on bitterly cold days—or for navigating sidewalks that are wet, icy, or slushy—you may want more rugged footwear such as hiking shoes. One place to look for these is at a sporting goods store. Hiking shoes have heavy-duty soles that grip better on sloppy or uneven terrain. They have elevated foot beds (because of the thickness of the soles), so your feet are higher than the water or slush that you're walking through. They're often waterproof, or at least water-resistant. And their tough exteriors stand up to the elements better than the average walking shoes.

A pair of hiking shoes made for trekking dirt trails should provide enough flexibility for fitness walking. And if you're expecting to end up with a pair of big, clunky "stompers," you're in for a pleasant surprise. These days, you can choose from lots of low-cut styles that are very lightweight and comfortable. (To get a pair that fits well, follow the shoe-buying guidelines in Chapter 8.)

If despite your best efforts your feet get cold and wet, handle them with care. "People with diabetes should be careful when walking in cold weather," says John M. Giurini, DPM, president-elect of the American College of Foot and Ankle Surgeons and associate professor in surgery at Harvard Medical School in Boston. "When you get home wash and dry your feet carefully. If you need to warm them up, do so gradually. If you dunk cold feet into hot water, they can get burned."

SHOW OFF YOUR SKIN SMARTS

When you're walking in wintry conditions, protecting your skin is very important, too. Cold and wind are no kinder than heat and sun. All can be quite drying. And don't let the chilly temperature fool you: The winter sun has ultraviolet rays that are strong enough to cause sunburn, age your skin, and increase your risk of skin cancer.

During the winter months, your hands and face are most vulnerable to the elements. You may wear gloves, only to have your hands get all sweaty as they warm up. But if you take off your gloves and expose your wet hands to the cold air, they may become chapped. That's why you should wear two pairs of gloves: thick ones on top, thin ones underneath. Leave on the thick pair until your hands feel warm, then slip them off and wear only the thin pair to protect your skin.

To save your face from the effects of wind and cold, invest in a ski mask. A thin one made from silk might be most comfortable, but check what's available. New, lightweight fabrics keep popping up everywhere.

If wearing a ski mask irritates your skin or obstructs your vision, you can go without one. But do wear a hat to keep body heat from escaping through the top of your head. To protect your face from the elements, first apply sunscreen and allow it to dry. Then add a thick layer of a protective moisturizer, petroleum jelly, or hand cream. Choose a sunscreen that's waterproof with an SPF of at least 15. Be sure to reapply both layers if you sweat a lot or wipe your face frequently.

If there's snow on the ground, you

need to be extra-vigilant about your sunscreen use. Snow reflects 85 percent of the sun's harmful ultraviolet rays right back at you, nearly doubling your exposure. The average person gets about 19 hours of sun each week, regardless of the season. That exposure accumulates from routine activities, such as walking your dog and driving a car. (UVA rays can penetrate most windows.)

According to one dermatologist, if you don't wear sunscreen between September and May, the damage to your skin could be the same as if you spent about eight straight summer weekends on the beach. Unfortunately, while 52 percent of Americans wear sunscreen in the summer, only 2 percent bother to slather it on in the winter. So here's your chance to do something good for your skin.

CHAPTER 14

EXERCISING IN
THE SNEEZIN' SEASON

According to the National Center for Health Statistics, more than 8 percent of Americans have what doctors call seasonal allergic rhinitis. The rest of us know it as hay fever.

If you're among the sniffling, sneezing millions, you already know that hay fever can wreak havoc on your walking program. In general, hay fever symptoms are most severe between August and October. That's when the big pollen producers, such as ragweed, pigweed, and lamb's-quarter, are in full bloom over most of the country. Mold spores are also especially troublesome in August, when their levels, spurred by summer rains, tend to peak. Between them, pollen and mold spores account for most cases of hay fever.

So what can you do to stifle your allergy symptoms, short of giving up walking until the first frost? Plenty, as it turns out. But you need to find out *exactly* what's causing your allergies before you can take steps to keep your walks symptom free.

THE SOURCE OF YOUR SYMPTOMS

If you've never been to an allergist, schedule an appointment with one. An allergist can perform skin tests to determine exactly which substances, or *allergens*, are triggering your symptoms. Once you know the specific offenders, you can plan your walking program so that you avoid them. Be sure to tell your allergist about your diabetes and any medications you're taking; this will be taken into account when treatments are prescribed.

If you're allergic to weed pollen, for example, you'll feel more comfortable if you do your walking later in the day. That's because weeds typically release their pollen early in the morning. And if you're allergic to molds, you'll be better off walking immediately after a rain. You have a window of a few hours from the time everything gets wet to the time the molds start producing spores like crazy.

Heavy rains also help people with pollen allergies by washing away pollen, but light rains actually make things worse. They break large clumps of pollen into tiny particles, which tend to remain airborne longer.

If rescheduling your walks is difficult or doesn't reduce your allergy symptoms as much as you'd like, then you may want to try premedication—that is, taking medicine before you go outdoors. An over-the-counter antihistamine may be enough to keep you walking right through allergy season. Your doctor or pharmacist can help you choose the one

that's right for you, taking care that it doesn't cause an interaction with any diabetes medications you may be taking.

Antihistamines are preventive medications. So for maximum effectiveness, they should be taken a half hour before you go walking. Some antihistamines can cause drowsiness or jitters. You may be able to minimize or avoid these side effects by starting at one-quarter to one-half the recommended dosage and taking a little more every day, working up to the full dosage over the course of 3 to 4 days.

If an over-the-counter drug doesn't do the trick, you may want to talk to your doctor about prescription-strength antihistamines. They're available in several forms, including pills, eyedrops that relieve itchy eyes, and nasal sprays that prevent allergy-induced stuffy noses.

Depending on the severity of your symptoms, you may even want to try allergy shots. You must get the shots year-round. Discuss them with your doctor to find out whether they'd be right for you.

TIPS FOR AVOIDING ALLERGENS

Whether or not you go the medication route, you have plenty of other options

Give Hypnosis a Whirl

If you're open to alternative therapies, try using your mind to manage your allergy symptoms. A handful of studies have found that, for some people, hypnosis provides relief.

Does this mean that allergies are all in your head? Not at all. But the study results provide additional evidence that the mind has greater influence over the body and physical responses than anyone ever imagined.

To find a health professional who's trained in medical hypnosis, visit the Web site of the American Society of Clinical Hypnosis, www.asch.net, or call them at 630-980-4740.

for reducing your exposure to allergens while you're walking. Here's what some experts recommend.

Keep tabs on the pollen count. You can get daily readings on pollen and mold levels from newspaper, radio, and TV weather forecasts, as well as from the Internet. If they're predicting a bad day, consider moving your walk indoors. Work out on a treadmill or head for a mall, where you can walk in climate-controlled, pollen-free comfort.

Pay attention to pollution. A number of studies have shown that if you're exposed to air pollution, especially ozone, you become sensitive to lower levels of airborne allergens. No one knows why, but scientists suspect that pollutants irritate the lining of the respiratory tract. So keep an ear to the news. If there's a pollution alert, plan on working out indoors that day. If you're on allergy medication, you may want to talk to your doctor about increasing your dosage when pollutant levels are high.

Steer clear of trouble spots. Plants that give off pollen tend to proliferate in vacant lots and other areas that aren't mowed regularly. To reduce your pollen exposure, you may have to find another route.

Warm up inside. If you stretch before you walk (and you should), plan to do your exercises indoors. That way, you spend less time out among the allergens. And the shorter your exposure to pollen or mold, the less severe your reaction will be.

Wear cool shades. Itchy, burning eyes are a hallmark of seasonal allergies. To keep pollen away from your eyes while you're walking, wear sunglasses. The bigger the glasses, the better their coverage. Wraparound and goggle-like styles are the best, because they cover more of the eye area. As a bonus, they block sun glare from the sides, so you can see where you're going.

Strap on a dust mask. If your allergy symptoms are really bothersome, you may not mind looking like Dr. Kildare. A dusk mask offers some protection by filtering out pollen. Look for the kind that are designed for industrial workers and home renovators. They're available in hardware stores and home centers.

Clean up after your workout. By showering and shampooing after your walk, you can remove most of the pollen that you picked up while outside. If you can't fit a shower into your schedule, at least wash your hands and face.

Sneeze-Free Walking Trips

If you have allergies and you're planning a walking vacation, you need to do some extra planning ahead. After all, you don't want to be caught unprepared in case your travel destination is in peak pollen season.

To get pollen and mold spore reports for locations throughout the United States, visit the www.aaaai.org/nab. This site, which is operated by the National Allergy Bureau of the American Academy of Allergy, Asthma and Immunology, provides regional pollen and mold spore counts.

PART IV

WALK OFF YOUR WEIGHT

CHAPTER 15

PICK YOUR PERSONAL SHAPE-UP PLAN

If you have diabetes, there's a good chance you could stand to lose a few pounds. People who are overweight are at the greatest risk for diabetes, and nearly 9 out of 10 people—90 percent!—with newly diagnosed type 2 diabetes are overweight. The good news is that losing some weight could help you manage your diabetes better.

"Losing weight can decrease insulin resistance," says Kashif Munir, MD, medical director of the Joslin Diabetes Center at Baltimore Washington Medical Center in Glen Burnie, Maryland. "In one study of patients with strong risk factors for developing diabetes, they found that the combination of diet and exercise was more effective than drugs to reduce the risk of developing diabetes. They divided the people into two groups. The first group ate a low-fat, low-calorie diet and did the equivalent of walking 30 minutes a day, 5 days per week, with the goal of losing 7 percent of their body weight. The other group took medication. After 3 years, the diet-and-exercise group had a 58 percent reduction in their risk of developing diabetes, compared with 31 percent for the medication group. Interestingly, people older than 60 in the diet-and-exercise group had a 71 percent reduction in risk."

So you have the will to lose the weight. Now you need the way. It's as simple as diet and exercise: They're the foundation of any sensible, successful weight loss program. Whether you want to shed 5 pounds or 50, the only surefire way to slim down is to use up more calories through regular physical activity than you take in from food.

And one of the best all-around activities for weight loss is—you guessed it—walking.

Never Too Busy for Exercise

Many fitness experts offer the same advice: To lose weight and get in shape, you must walk for an hour a day at least 5 days a week. That's 1 hour. Sixty whole minutes.

That sure seems like a big chunk out of a short day. In fact, setting aside an hour for exercise can so overwhelm people that they give up on slimming down. But here's a simple solution: Divvy up that hour over the course of a day.

That's right. While some people were insisting that anything less than an hour of exercise wouldn't cut the fat, researchers discovered that little bits of activity squeezed in throughout the day were just as good as one big chunk—and maybe even better.

Think about how you can break down your walking routine. If a 1-hour walk every morning is difficult, cut back to a short, 20-minute a.m. workout. That done, you've fulfilled one-third of your daily walking requirement.

At lunchtime, eat something light, then step out for a brisk walk. Twenty minutes is plenty. For the day, it's 40 minutes down, 20 to go.

Those last 20 minutes likely present the biggest challenge. You could take a short walking break in the afternoon or a lap around the block before your drive home from work, or take a quick spin on the treadmill once you get home.

The latest research suggests that short bursts of activity may cause your body to burn calories more steadily throughout the day. Seems that "incremental exercise" is an idea whose time has come.

Granted, other forms of exercise—such as running, bicycling, and swimming—may burn more calories per minute. But studies have shown that people who take up walking actually stick with it, while those who pursue other activities tend to give up after the first few months. What's more, walking is gentle and low impact, a plus if you've been sedentary for a while. And it's easy to incorporate into your daily routine. No packing a bag and driving to the gym.

This chapter features three basic programs for beginning to experienced walkers. Just read through the plans—the Get-Started Plan on page 106, the Plateau-Busting Plan on page 107, and the Maximum-Calorie-Burn Plan on page 109—and choose the one that best matches your current fitness level, lifestyle, and weight loss goals.

After 4 weeks of walking (the duration of each plan), you should notice the pounds melting away. How fast they disappear varies from one person to the next. If you're more than 50 pounds overweight and you've been sedentary for years, you may start losing almost immediately. If you've been losing but seem be stuck at a certain number, you may need a bit more time to see results.

Remember, too, that the goal of walking is to get fit and healthy, not to be pencil-thin. Even losing 10 percent of your body weight can cut your risk of serious illness. Every step you take reduces stress and boosts your energy level. And that's definitely something to stride for.

THE GET-STARTED PLAN

Choose this beginning-level program if any of the following applies.

- You're severely overweight.
- You're recovering from illness or surgery.
- You have a chronic health problem that limits activity.
- You devote less than 60 minutes a day to "active" tasks like walking the dog, chasing after kids, or putting out the garbage.
- You spend your days sitting at a desk or in your car and your evenings lounging on the couch.

With the Get-Started Plan, you'll ease your way into a regular walking routine. It starts you out slowly, to build your confidence and reduce your risk of injury. Even at a moderate pace, you'll reap many benefits. ("Moderate" means you're moving fast enough to get your heart pumping but not so fast that you become out of breath.) Almost immediately, you'll notice improvements in your flexibility, your energy level, and your mood. After the second week of the program, your workouts will feel easier—a sign that your heart is getting fitter and your legs are getting stronger.

The Get-Started Plan

During week 1 of this program, walk at a speed that feels comfortable for you. Then in weeks 2 through 4, pick up your pace a bit, as though you're in a hurry to get somewhere.

WEEK	DURATION (MIN.)	FREQUENCY (DAYS/WEEK)	INTENSITY
1	10	3	Moderate
2	15	4	Moderate
3	20	5	Moderate
4	30	5	Moderate

THE PLATEAU-BUSTING PLAN

If you agree with any of these statements, this program is perfect for you.

• Your scale hasn't budged for the past month.
• You've been walking regularly for at least 6 weeks.
• You're bored with walking, and you're starting to skip workouts.
• You don't have a formal exercise routine, but your days are active.

As its name suggests, the Plateau-Busting Plan is designed to jump-start a weight loss regimen that has stalled. Sometimes a simple change in your workout is all you need to start shedding pounds again. It not only increases your calorie burn but also breathes new life into your workouts—a great way to combat boredom.

In the chart on page 108, you'll see the phrase "rate of perceived exertion." It refers to the Borg Rating of Perceived Exertion (RPE) Scale (see below), an easy method of assessing how hard you're exercising.

Borg Rating of Perceived Exertion Scale

6	Very, very light (lounging on the couch)
7	
8	
9	Very light (puttering around the house)
10	
11	Fairly light (strolling leisurely)
12	
13	Somewhat hard (walking normally)
14	
15	Hard (walking as if in a hurry)
16	
17	Very hard (jogging or running)
18	
19	Very, very hard (sprinting)
20	

The Plateau-Busting Plan

This plan uses intervals—periods of brisk walking, followed by periods of recovery—to step up calorie burn and send those stubborn pounds packing.

WEEK	PROGRAM	RATE OF PERCEIVED EXERTION
1: Exercise for 35 minutes, 5 days this week.	Warmup (5 min.)	10–11
	Normal walk (5 min.)	13
	Speed-up (5 min.)	15
	Recover (10 min.)	13
	Speed-up (5 min.)	15
	Cooldown (5 min.)	10–11
2: Exercise for 35 minutes, 5 days this week.	Warmup (5 min.)	10–11
	Normal walk (5 min.)	13
	Speed-up (5 min.)	16
	Recover (10 min.)	13
	Speed-up (5 min.)	16
	Cooldown (5 min.)	10–11

To use RPE, do a mental scan of your body while you're walking. Is your breathing heavy? Are you sweating? Do your muscles feel warm? Are they burning? Based on your scan, rate your walk on the Borg scale.

Quick Tip

If you're just beginning a walking program, choose a route that takes you in a short loop, so you're never too far from your house or car if you get tired. People with heart or respiratory conditions might even start out by walking to the end of their driveways and back, over and over, to build up their endurance.

WEEK	PROGRAM	RATE OF PERCEIVED EXERTION
3: Exercise for 45 minutes, 5 days this week.	Warmup (5 min.)	10–11
	Normal walk (5 min.)	13
	Speed-up (5 min.)	16
	Recover (8 min.)	13
	Speed-up (5 min.)	16
	Recover (7 min.)	13
	Speed-up (5 min.)	16
	Cooldown (5 min.)	10–11
4: Exercise for 45 minutes, 5 days this week.	Warmup (5 min.)	10–11
	Speed-up (5 min.)	16
	Recover (5 min.)	13
	Speed-up (5 min.)	16
	Recover (5 min.)	13
	Speed-up (5 min.)	16
	Recover (5 min.)	13
	Speed-up (5 min.)	16
	Cooldown (5 min.)	10–11

THE MAXIMUM-CALORIE-BURN PLAN

Do any of these statements describe you? If so, then this is your program.

- You think walking is too easy.
- You want to lose weight fast.
- You've been doing intervals—periods of brisk walking, followed by periods of recovery—for at least 6 weeks.
- You don't have time for longer walks.

In the Maximum-Calorie-Burn Plan, you'll be doing what's called a Power Pyramid. Basically, you work your way up to a brief but very high-intensity walk or jog, then work your way back down. To make the intervals easier, you might want to record some favorite upbeat tunes and add voice cues every 30 to 60 seconds to indicate when to change pace. That sure beats constantly checking your watch.

The Maximum-Calorie-Burn Plan

This workout features Power Pyramids, which pump up the intensity and, therefore, the calorie-burning capacity of your walking program. To do a pyramid, simply follow the instructions in the graph below.

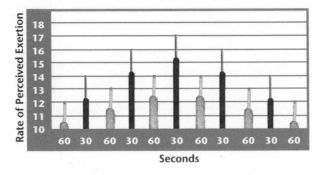

This graph shows you how to do a Power Pyramid. The numbers across the bottom indicate the length of each mini-interval, while the numbers on the left-hand side represent rate of perceived exertion (RPE). So for the first interval, which lasts 60 seconds, your RPE should be 12. When you complete one interval, move on to the next until you've worked through all of them. Then refer to the chart below.

WEEK	PROGRAM	RATE OF PERCEIVED EXERTION
1: Exercise for approximately 40 minutes, 5 days this week.	Warmup (5 min.)	10–11
	Pyramid	See graph
	Normal walk (7 min.)	13
	Pyramid	See graph
	Normal walk (6 min.)	13
	Cooldown (5 min.)	10–11

WEEK	PROGRAM	RATE OF PERCEIVED EXERTION
2: Exercise for approximately 45 minutes, 5 days this week.	Warmup (5 min.)	10–11
	Pyramid	See graph
	Normal walk (5 min.)	13
	Pyramid	See graph
	Normal walk (5 min.)	13
	Pyramid	See graph
	Cooldown (5 min.)	10–11
3: Exercise for approximately 50 minutes, 5 days this week.	Warmup (5 min.)	10–11
	Pyramid	See graph
	Normal walk (5 min.)	13
	Pyramid	See graph
	Normal walk (5 min.)	13
	Pyramid	See graph
	Normal walk (5 min.)	13
	Cooldown (5 min.)	10–11
4: Exercise for approximately 60 minutes, 5 days this week.	Warmup (5 min.)	10–11
	Pyramid	See graph
	Normal walk (5 min.)	13
	Pyramid	See graph
	Normal walk (5 min.)	13
	Pyramid	See graph
	Normal walk (5 min.)	13
	Pyramid	See graph
	Cooldown (5 min.)	10–11

CHAPTER 16

REV UP YOUR WARMUP

We know why you always skip the 5-minute warmup that experts insist upon: It's borrrinnng. Besides, when you have scarcely 30 minutes slotted for exercise in a time-crunched schedule, you don't want to waste even one valuable fat-blasting, butt-firming minute doing tedious in-place marches and shoulder rolls.

"Warming up is important because it prevents injury and makes exercise feel easier, but it doesn't have to be dull," says Fabio Comana, an ACE-certified personal trainer and an exercise physiology instructor at the University of California, San Diego. With Comana's help, we've tweaked the tired, same-old warmup to create a batch of fresh moves that will make your opening act rock.

This routine features dynamic drills such as the Back Twist, which warms and stretches your body, along with balance and agility exercises to bolster core strength, stability, and overall coordination—skills that often get short shrift in a regular workout, says Comana. Do the following preworkout prep for 5 to 10 minutes before your regular cardio or strength-training workout. No time for a real workout? Do a second set of all the warmup moves and you'll have a quick, stand-alone total-body routine.

STEP-HOP AND KICK

Warms glutes, hamstrings, quads, calves, and shoulders

STAND with your feet hip-width apart and your elbows bent at 90 degrees. Step forward with your right leg, and as your right foot touches the floor, push up onto the ball of your foot with a hop, bring your left knee up to hip height, and swing your right arm forward (pictured). Lower your left leg and repeat, alternating legs as you step-hop for 30 seconds. (Always keep one foot on the floor.) Continue step-hopping, but when your knee comes up, kick that leg out, toe pointed. Alternate legs for 30 seconds.

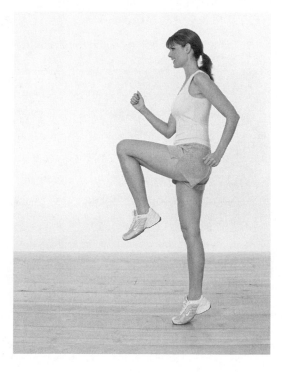

ROTATING LUNGE

Builds balance, stability, and core strength

STAND with your feet hip-width apart, holding a pillow at chest level. Take a giant step forward with your left leg. Bend your left knee and lower until your thigh is parallel with the floor. Hold, and rotate your torso to the right for 2 seconds, keeping the pillow in front of your chest (pictured). Rotate to the center and then stand back up, bringing your right foot next to your left. Repeat, stepping with your right leg and twisting to your left. Alternate for 10 to 12 reps each side.

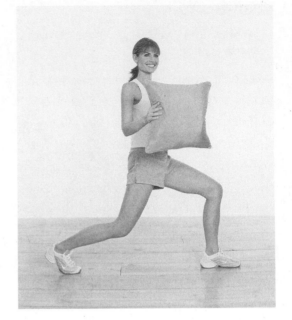

STORK FLY

Improves posture, balance, core stability, and strength

STAND with your feet together and extend your arms to shoulder height, with your palms facing up. Raise your left knee so your thigh is almost parallel with the floor. Keep your hips level. Hold for 10 to 15 seconds.

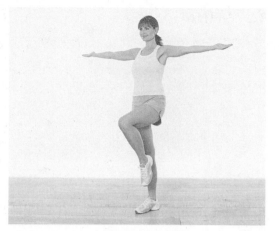

WITH your left knee lifted, bend your torso forward, extend your left leg back, and raise your arms overhead until your arms, torso, and left leg are parallel to floor. Hold for 10 to 15 seconds, then slowly return to start. Switch legs and repeat.

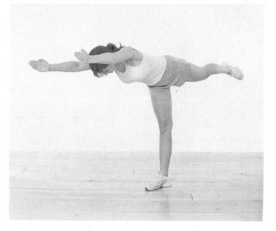

PILLOW THROW

Develops agility, coordination, balance, core stability, and strength

BALANCE on your right leg. Hold a small pillow in your left hand, with your right arm out for balance.

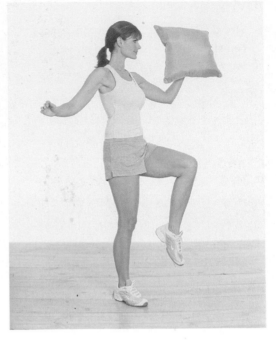

As if pitching a baseball in slow motion, rotate your torso and left arm in a downward diagonal arc, follow the pillow with your eyes, and swing your left leg down and back without touching the floor. Hold for 1 to 2 seconds. Reverse the action to slowly come back up. Switch sides and repeat. Too difficult? Try the move looking straight ahead or with both feet on floor. Alternate for 8 to 10 reps on each side.

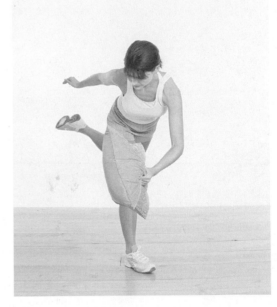

BACK TWIST

Stretches and warms glutes, hip flexors, hamstrings, lower back, and core rotating muscles

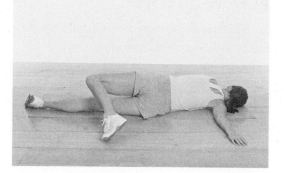

LIE facedown with your legs straight and your arms extended out to your sides, palms down. Bend your left knee and rotate your left hip and leg up and over your back until your left foot touches the floor on the right side. Keep your upper body and right hip and leg on the floor (pictured). Return to start and repeat with the right leg. Alternate for 8 to 10 reps on each side, holding each move for 1 to 2 seconds.

TOUCH-DOWN

Warms inner and outer thighs and lower-back muscles; strengthens core

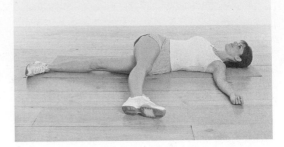

LIE faceup with your arms out to your sides. Raise your right leg so it's perpendicular to the floor. Lower your right leg across your torso and touch the floor on your left side with your right foot (pictured). Return to start; do 8 to 10 reps. Repeat with your left leg. (This exercise is not recommended for people with back problems.)

Warmup 101

Here's why you need it:

For a kick: Warming up increases your energy and endurance by supplying your muscles with more oxygen.

To boost your burn: These moves mimic the patterns in cardio and strength routines, which means your muscles will fire faster and work harder during exercise.

To stay the course: Don't become another "I used to work out until I pulled my back" statistic. These exercises will improve your range of motion by increasing bloodflow and muscle temperature, reducing your risk of injury.

CHAPTER 17

WALK THE WEIGHT OFF—ANYWHERE

Get ready to be inspired: This workout trio may just make winter your favorite walking season. Head outdoors for a routine that cranks up the intensity, helps keep your muscles warm, and ensures a quick return home. If getting outside is impossible, we've also provided an at-home treadmill workout. We even have a fitness walk you can do while shopping at the mall! "The more options you have, the more likely you'll be to stick to an exercise routine, no matter what the weather," says certified personal trainer Kate Larsen, author of *Progress Not Perfection: Your Journey Matters*. Keep up the hard work all season long, and by spring, you might be shopping for a smaller size!

Pace Yourself for Best Results

Here are the pace and exertion levels you'll find in these workouts:

Easy: You can sing.
Moderate: You can talk freely.
Brisk: You can talk but you'd rather not.
Fast: You're huffing and puffing.
Sprint: You can't go for longer than 30 seconds.

Mall Moves

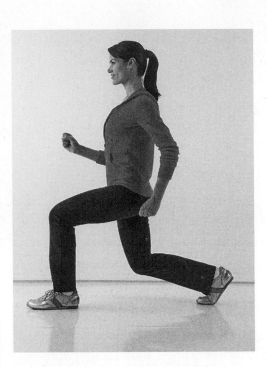

Walking Lunge: Step your left foot forward about 3 feet, letting your arms swing naturally. Bend your left knee until your left thigh is nearly parallel with the floor and your right thigh is near the floor. Keep your left knee over your ankle and your abs tight. Stand, bringing your right foot next to your left one. Then step your right foot forward and repeat.

Bench Pushup: Place your hands shoulder-width apart on the back of a bench or railing. Walk your feet back so your body forms a diagonal line. Bend your elbows and lower your chest toward the bench. Hold for one count, then straighten your arms.

Squat Walk-Up: Stand facing a staircase with your feet together. Place your right foot on the second step and bend your knees, sitting back into a squat. Climb the stairs two at a time, maintaining the squat position as much as possible. Hold on to the railing for safety.

Stair Hops: Stand facing a staircase with your feet together. Hop onto the first step, landing with your knees bent. Step backward off of the step, one foot at a time. Repeat, hopping onto the bottom step and stepping off of it, alternating feet.

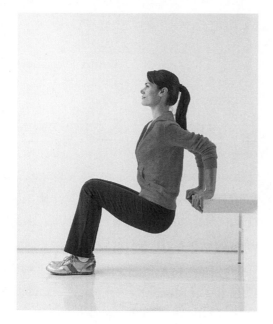

Triceps Dips: Sit on the edge of a bench with your hands next to your hips, grasping the seat edge. Slide your butt off of the bench and walk your feet forward so your knees are over your ankles. Lower your butt toward the floor, bending your elbows up to 90 degrees. Keep your elbows pointing behind you. Hold for one count, then straighten your arms.

HOP ON THE TREADMILL

This hill-heavy routine sculpts and strengthens thighs and glutes, says creator Jennifer Renfroe, group fitness coordinator and a treadmill class instructor at Crunch Gym in Atlanta. "Feel free to adjust the speed and incline depending on your personal fitness level," she advises.

What you'll need: A treadmill with an incline adjustment

The Routine:

Duration: 45 minutes

0–2:00 Easy walk (warmup)

2:01–5:00 Moderate walk

5:01–10:00 Hill drill: Brisk walk, increasing incline one level every minute

10:01–12:00 Lower incline to level 1 and walk briskly

12:01–17:00 Hill drill: Brisk walk, increasing speed by 0.1 mph and incline by one level every minute

17:01–19:00 Lower incline to level 2 and walk at a moderate pace

19:01–20:00 Raise incline to level 5 and walk briskly

20:01–24:00 Hill drill: Brisk walk, increasing speed by 0.1 mph and incline by one level every minute

24:01–26:00 Lower incline to level 2 and walk at a moderate pace

26:01–40:00 Repeat minutes 19:01–26:00 two times

40:01–45:00 Easy walk, return incline to level 1 (cooldown)

Boost your burn: Strap on a PowerBelt (about $75 at www.walkerswarehouse.com), a lightweight padded belt that's equipped with retractable resistance cords, and give your upper body a workout. Hold the cords while you swing your arms forward, backward, up, or down and you'll burn as much as 64 percent more calories.

HIT THE MALL

Many shopping malls open early for walkers, and some, like Minnesota's Mall of America, even have walking clubs. (Contact malls in your area to find a club near you.)

What you'll need: Your usual walking gear—even shorts if you want

The Routine:

Duration: 1 hour

0–2:00 Easy walk (warmup)

2:01–4:00 Moderate walk

4:01–10:00 Brisk walk

10:01–30:00 Fast walk

30:01–33:00 Walking Lunges

33:01–35:00 Bench Pushups

35:01–45:00 Fast walk

45:01–47:00 Squat Walk-Ups

47:01–49:00 Stair Hops

49:01–51:00 Triceps Dips

51:01–57:00 Brisk walk

57:01–60:00 Easy walk (cooldown)

Boost your burn: Wear a weighted vest (about $130 at www.x2vest.com) that allows you to add small weights to your core. For each additional 5 pounds you carry, you'll burn about 5 percent more calories and tone up faster. Skip the ankle and hand weights, says Larsen, who developed this workout. They put undue stress on those injury-prone joints.

GET OUTSIDE

"The jumping and sprinting in this workout really challenge muscles, providing additional sculpting," says Therese Iknoian, a California-based exercise physiologist, author of *Fitness Walking*, and creator of this workout. The built-in bonus of braving the cold: You burn calories just staying warm.

What you'll need: Essential winter gear (see tips below)

Essential Winter Wear

On the bottom: A fabric like Coolmax that wicks away sweat

Middle: An insulating fleece such as Polartec

Top: Something wind-resistant and waterproof, like Gore-Tex

Shoes: Water-resistant and warm with slip-proof treaded or lug soles

Hat and gloves: Soft fleece fabrics that won't itch or chafe against your skin

The Routine:

Duration: 30 minutes

0–2:00 Easy walk (warmup)

2:01–4:00 Moderate walk, lifting knees for 60 seconds, then circling arms backward (30 seconds) and forward (30 seconds)

4:01–7:00 Brisk walk

7:01–8:00 Climb stairs or step off and onto a curb

8:01–9:00 Do pushups against a tree, bench, or other sturdy object

9:01–9:30 Bend knees and jump to touch overhead branch or sign; repeat

9:31–11:00 Brisk walk

11:01–15:00 Repeat minutes 7:01–11:00

15:01–25:00 Alternate fast walking and sprinting to landmarks located 50 yards apart (about half a football field)

25:01–28:00 Brisk walk

28:01–30:00 Easy walk (cooldown)

Boost your burn: Walking in snowshoes blasts twice as many calories; walking poles (about $100 at www.walkingpoles.com), about 20 percent more.

Walk It Off at Home!

Try *Prevention* magazine's exercise DVD *Walk Yourself Fit* for three more indoor walking routines that burn fat. You can order it at www.preventionfitness.com.

CHAPTER 18

WHAT'S THE SPEED FOR SLIMMING DOWN?

A few years back, long slow distance was all the rage for weight loss. Why? Because a few studies suggested that walking at a comfortable, moderate pace helps the body preferentially burn fat. For weight-conscious walkers, the mantra became "Slow down!" Going too fast uses up carbohydrates but not fat stores.

At first, the advice seemed to defy logic. After all, most of us were convinced that exercising hard *must* get rid of more fat by burning more calories. But perhaps because this new fitness philosophy meant that we didn't have to sweat to slim down, it went over big.

The fact is, as long as you use up more calories through physical activity than you take in from food, you'll lose fat and weight in the long run. Whether that physical activity is slow or fast doesn't really matter. At any speed, *calories burned are calories burned*.

FASTER IS BETTER . . . SOMETIMES

Of course, not everyone loses weight at the same rate. You probably know people who shed pounds like a duck's feathers shed water. They were inactive for years, yet ever since they started exercising, the fat has just melted away.

Other people—and maybe you're one of them—have worked out religiously for years. Even though they're in better shape and they feel great, the number on the scale has hardly budged. Obviously, these folks need to do something differently if they want to slim down. But does that mean they need to *slow* down?

Calories Go, Fast or Slow

The chart below, adapted from *Sports Nutrition for the '90s* by Jacqueline Berning, RD, and Suzanne Nelson Steen, RD, compares the number of calories burned by an average 150-pound person while walking at various speeds. As you can see, the faster you go, the more calories you use per minute. But if you figure out the number of calories burned per mile, there's not that much difference between walking slow and walking fast.

For example, a 20-minute-per-mile pace burns 4.1 calories per minute, or 82 calories per mile ($20 \times 4.1 = 82$). By comparison, a 12-minute-per-mile pace burns 8.2 calories per minute, or 98.4 calories per mile ($12 \times 8.2 = 98.4$). That's just 16 calories more—and you can easily make up for that by walking an extra $\frac{1}{4}$ mile at the slower pace.

So if you're walking to lose weight, remember that you don't need to push yourself at top speed. Going slower but farther—long slow distance—can produce the same results.

SPEED (MPH)	MINUTES PER MILE	CALORIES BURNED PER MINUTE
1.0	60.0	2.3
2.0	30.0	3.2
2.3	26.0	3.5
3.0	20.0	4.1
3.2	18.5	4.7
3.5	17.1	5.1
4.0	15.0	6.4
4.5	13.2	7.1
5.0	12.0	8.2

Well, at least one study seems to challenge the long slow distance theory. Researchers at West Virginia University in Morgantown recruited two groups of volunteers—one to work out at a high intensity, the other at a moderate intensity. Both groups exercised for the same amount of time and the same number of days every week. Neither was asked to follow any specific dietary guidelines.

Over the 11 weeks of the study, the high-intensity exercisers reduced their body fat and improved their cardiovascular conditioning, while the moderate-intensity exercisers showed no changes. Interestingly, the high-intensity exercisers reported that they automatically began eating less saturated fat and more carbohydrates. Apparently, their bodies naturally craved carbs for quick energy.

Does this mean that you *should* work out at a high intensity—that's 80 to 90 percent of your maximum heart rate—if you want to lose weight? (To find your maximum heart rate, subtract your age from 220.) "There do seem to be some advantages to working at high intensities," notes Randall W. Byrne, EdD, who led the study. "But there's no advantage if you hate walking fast and stop exercising altogether. Besides, for some people, such as those with heart disease, diabe-

tes, or asthma, high-intensity exercise may not be safe."

One other point worth making: This study lasted just 11 weeks, a relatively short time in which to bring about weight loss through physical activity alone. In a longer trial, both groups may have shed pounds without altering their eating habits.

MAKING A CASE FOR A MODERATE PACE

While brisk walking and long slow distance may have the same calorie- and fat-burning capacity over the long run, long slow distance has other advantages that may make it a better choice for you. For example, maybe you feel that sweaty, heart-pounding workouts should be reserved for Olympians and professional athletes. Or perhaps your physical condition makes brisk walking difficult, if not impossible. Or maybe you're the sort of person who would rather walk 5 miles at a moderate pace than racewalk around the block.

All of these are perfectly legitimate reasons to opt for long slow distance. Just remember that the slower your pace, the farther you need to go to burn the same number of calories that you would at a fast pace—hence the phrase "long slow distance." Makes sense, right?

Many fitness experts swear by long slow distance. Among them is Rob Sweetgall, who has written a number of books on walking. He also created the Walking Wellness school curriculum, which helps teachers develop lesson plans that encourage kids to learn about their bodies and explore the world through walking.

Sweetgall became an expert on walking by . . . well, walking. In fact, he has trekked across the country seven times, including an 11,208-mile excursion that took him to all 50 states and lasted an entire year.

With almost two decades of walking experience to back him up, Sweetgall maintains that a moderate pace is the best pace for anyone at any age. "I'm convinced that the human body is a $3^1/_2$-mile-per-hour walking machine," he says. "Even slowing down from 4 miles per hour to $3^1/_2$ is better for most people. I've walked across America at both speeds, and I had much less soreness at the slower pace. Personally, I'd rather enjoy walking and *not* get sore."

Sweetgall believes that the purpose of walking is to keep yourself healthy and functional, so you can enjoy life to the fullest. You don't need to go fast to expe-rience those benefits. "Of the thousands of people who attend my workshops, those who have the most aches and pains are almost always pushing them-selves, trying to go a few gears higher," he says. "Don't get me wrong—I myself engage in intense exercise from time to time. But I can reach my target heart rate at just 2 miles per hour by Exerstrid-ing [walking with special fitness poles] up a steep hill or climbing a ridge near my home in snowshoes."

What about walking for weight loss? Sweetgall still thinks distance is more important than speed. The more dis-tance you cover, he reasons, the more calories you're going to burn. "If you increase from a 17-minute mile to a 15-minute mile, you may use 9 percent more calories per mile. If you double your distance, you use 100 percent more calories. That's why I tell people to walk at their most comfortable pace and to stop worrying about whether they're going fast enough."

Ultimately, whether you choose brisk walking or long slow distance depends on your fitness level and your personal pref-erences. Do what feels right for you. And if your goal is to lose weight, know that you don't need to speedwalk to see results. Slow and steady sheds pounds, too.

In Step with Dick Barr

He Had to Slow Down to Slim Down

Dick "The Bear" Barr spent years trying to walk off some extra weight. But no matter how many miles he logged, he couldn't seem to slim down. Then he changed his attitude toward exercise—and he easily dropped 75 pounds in 18 months.

A resident of Edmonton in Alberta, Canada, Dick never got a driver's license. He relied on his feet to take him where he wanted to go. Yet even though he walked everywhere, he was carrying 260 pounds on his 6-foot-1 frame.

Back then, Dick aimed for a certain number of miles. "I walked 8 to 10 miles a day, going to and from work—and I'd go out again *after* work," he recalls. "I rushed to get my miles in."

Unfortunately, Dick didn't realize that his high-gear approach to walking—and the hearty appetite that it produced—was undermining his efforts to slim down. In fact, over the next 10 years, his weight crept up to 284 pounds.

That's when he set out to do things a little differently. "I decided that my rushed way of walking was for the birds," he says. "I kept on walking, but I focused more on being healthy, as opposed to racking up miles. I threw out my bathroom scale because I didn't want the frustration of looking at the numbers every day."

Dick also began paying more attention to his eating habits. He ate only when he felt hungry, snacking on fruit in the middle of the day to tide him over until dinnertime. He slowed the pace of his meals so that he'd recognize when he was full and not stuff himself.

Dick's plan worked like a charm, as the pounds finally started melting away. "I was so surprised by how fast I lost weight that I went to my doctor just to make sure everything was okay," he says. "He told me that I was in great shape—and to keep walking!"

Dick remains an avid walker, only now he goes at a more leisurely pace. "I'm much more relaxed about it," he says. "And when I'm in a group, I've learned to love being at the back of the pack."

CHAPTER 19

GREAT GADGETS FOR BOOSTING YOUR BURN

Many people are drawn to walking for its purity. No special equipment, memberships, or fees are required. However, other people like gadgets in every shape and form, even when doing something as simple as walking.

Most walkers fall somewhere between the gadget leery and gadget loving. No matter where you fall on this spectrum, two gadgets are especially helpful and fun to use: the PowerBelt and walking poles.

PUMPING IRON WITHOUT THE IRON

The PowerBelt is a portable fitness machine that you wear around your waist, just like a belt. It has two handles that you hold while you walk, swinging your arms back and forth. (Surprisingly, you can move your arms in close-to-natural fitness-walking or racewalking form.) The handles are attached to cords, which are wound around spring-action disks. The disks provide resistance when you pull on the handles. This increases your heart rate, and it also tones the muscles in your shoulders, arms, and back.

Unlike hand weights, the PowerBelt doesn't strain your wrists. If your arms get tired, just let go of the handles. They pop right back into place on the belt. No need to lug them around. Once your arms have rested a bit, just grab the handles and start swinging.

The PowerBelt comes with special attachments, called PowerPaks, that progressively increase the resistance you feel when you pull on the handles. The PowerPaks can be added anytime, such as when you want to do intervals (periods of brisk walking followed by periods of recovery).

Actually, you don't need the Power-Paks to get a good workout. Researchers at the University of Wisconsin–La Crosse found that walking with the PowerBelt set at its lowest resistance burns 48 percent more calories than walking at the same speed without the belt. That's an impressive gain, even without the extra resistance.

While you walk, you can experiment with the handles, too. For example, you can give your shoulder and arm muscles more of a workout by pulling the handles out to the sides or up over your head. It's great for walking on treadmills, too.

The PowerBelt sells for about $75. You may be able to find it in a sporting goods or fitness equipment store. If not, you can order it online at www.walkerswarehouse.com.

USING POLES TO INCREASE INTENSITY

A former cross-country skier named Tom Rutlin developed a pair of walking poles that he called Exerstriders. Rutlin looks years younger than his chronological age, but he swears that he hasn't lifted

---

Another Plus for Poles

If you have osteoarthritis or another joint disease, or if you're on the mend from a knee injury, walking poles can help you ease into exercise by reducing the force of your footsteps. According to Michael Torry, PhD, of the Steadman-Hawkins Sports Medicine Foundation in Vail, Colorado, walking with poles can reduce the accumulated force by about 6 tons over the course of a mile. That way, you keep your workouts low impact and pain free.

a weight or used an exercise machine in 15 years. He attributes his trim waist and muscled arms and legs to walking with poles. "It allows me to work all of my muscles with one total-body activity," he explains.

Rutlin feels that total-body exercise such as walking with poles is the key to weight loss and overall fitness. It not only boosts aerobic capacity but also builds muscle strength and endurance. "Most people don't have time to do aerobic exercise *and* strength training," he explains. "Walking with poles combines both."

Swimming, rowing, and cross-country skiing are also forms of total-body exercise. But depending where you live, you can't do any of these activities year-round unless you have access to an indoor swimming pool or a rowing or cross-country ski machine. That's what makes walking with poles an ideal workout for so many people.

"Exerstriding [walking with poles] is a simple, safe, enjoyable activity that uses almost all of your muscles in a single exercise session," Rutlin says. "If done properly, it builds muscle in both your upper and lower body while providing enough of an aerobic workout to melt away fat. In fact, walking with poles burns 20 to 50 percent more calories than walking without poles at the same pace."

You might want to keep a pair of Exerstriders in the back of your car for spur-of-the-moment workouts. They're like having an extra pair of feet for support. They're also a nice piece of insurance, should you encounter any aggressive dogs on your walks.

The Exerstriders come with a booklet and a DVD or VHS video that show you stretching exercises you can do with the poles.

The Exerstrider walking poles cost $89.95 per pair. To order, visit www.exerstrider.com or call 800-554-0989. Either way, you'll need to specify your height, so you get the right-size poles. There is a 60-day return policy.

CHAPTER 20

A WALKER'S GUIDE TO EATING FOR WEIGHT LOSS

No doubt about it: Walking can do wonders for your body, helping you to stay fit and healthy. But if your goal is to slim down, walking is only part of the equation. You need to eat right, too.

Of course, eating right with diabetes is challenging enough. Eating right with diabetes and trying to lose weight is a whole other level of challenging. So what should you eat if you have diabetes?

"My best advice is to consult with a registered dietitian and construct a nutritious and heart-healthy Mediterranean-style diet plan—one that's rich in fruits, vegetables, whole grains, nuts, legumes, olive oil, and fish," says Janet Bond Brill, PhD, RD, LDN, nutritionist, exercise physiologist, and adjunct professor of nutrition, health, and fitness at the Robert Stempel School of Public Health at Florida International University in Miami. "I also recommend utilizing the American Diabetes Association Exchange Lists for Meal Planning to adjust food to insulin and insulin to food, based on carbohydrate counting and blood glucose levels."

SHEDDING POUNDS STARTS WITH YOUR PLATE

With those basics down, what should you do if you have diabetes and have to lose weight? One simple eating plan isn't really a plan at all. It doesn't

Eat Like a Weight Loss Winner

Why reinvent the wheel? Sometimes the best way to do something is doing what people who succeeded did.

"I always recommend that my patients learn the weight loss secrets of success from the true experts at weight loss, those people that have joined the National Weight Control Registry," says Janet Bond Brill, PhD, RD, LDN, nutritionist, exercise physiologist, and author of *Cholesterol Down*. "The National Weight Control Registry is a group of individuals who have done the impossible: lost a significant amount of weight *and kept it off*. Do what they did is my advice."

Here are four secrets of these weight loss winners.

Use a combination of diet plus exercise to lose weight. Registrants used a variety of methods to lose weight (50 percent on formal diets, 50 percent on their own), with both groups using a combination of diet and exercise for their initial weight loss. What they all have in common, however, are their similar behavioral strategies for maintaining the weight loss: They eat a nutritious calorie-

involve counting calories or calculating percentages of carbohydrates, protein, and fat. It's much simpler than that. You just need to redesign your dinner plate.

You've seen those paper plates that are divided into sections, right? If you were to use one of those to serve a typical American meal, the largest section—about half the plate—would be filled with meat. The other two sections would hold mostly fats and refined carbohydrates. Those proportions just don't fuel the body optimally.

In fact, we Americans eat some 839 *billion* calories of fat every year. That translates to about 35 percent of total calorie intake—a megadose compared with the 25 percent recommended by experts. And all that fat is leaving little

controlled diet, and they also eat healthfully consistently throughout the entire week rather than just dieting during weekdays.

Eat breakfast. Almost 80 percent of registrants eat breakfast daily.

Use frequent self-monitoring techniques to keep yourself on track. Weigh yourself at least once a week and keep a food and exercise diary, for example.

Exercise, exercise, exercise! The common thread running through all of the successful weight loss maintainers is their high level of physical activity, including moving around more in everyday life and getting in planned exercise sessions. Registrants average 60 to 90 minutes of physical activity daily, with walking being the most popular form of physical activity.

"The take-away message from the masters of weight control is that for a lifetime of weight management, you need to change your behavior pattern of eating and exercise, or lack thereof," says Dr. Brill. "You can't buy a magical weight loss bullet at the store. A lifetime of weight control involves focusing day-in and day-out on eating a healthy, low-calorie, balanced diet, and combining that way of eating with a highly active lifestyle."

room for nutrient-dense vegetables and other wholesome foods.

To trim your fat intake and create more balanced meals without measuring, just change the proportions on your plate. Going back to that divided paper plate, instead of putting the meat in the largest section, trim the portion so that it fits in one of the small sections. That's about a 3-ounce serving, roughly the size of a deck of playing cards, the amount considered healthy by nutrition experts.

As for the rest of the plate, fill the largest section with vegetables and the remaining small section with grains. Actually, you can let the grains spill over into the veggies if you want. And as you lose weight, you can adjust the portions even more, so the grains and vegetables are about equal. This increases your calorie intake a bit without adding on pounds.

Reconfiguring your dinner plate in this way makes healthy eating easy. It provides the right mix of nutrients while automatically slashing calories and grams of fat. And because your plate is full, the portions look adequate and appealing, so you won't feel deprived. That's key to making permanent changes in your eating habits.

To complement your healthy meals, use your snack times to nibble on your choice of fresh, juicy fruits. Try papayas, mangoes, kiwis, and other exotic options that you might normally pass by.

FILL UP, NOT OUT

Bet you didn't think eating for weight loss could be so simple. But it is! To keep meal preparation fast and your foods nutritious and tasty, just follow this advice.

For veggies, outsmart the seasons. Some vegetables—such as summer and winter squash, cabbage, lettuce, and tomatoes—taste best fresh. Most others are quite good frozen. So when fresh isn't available or convenient, reap the bounty of your supermarket's frozen foods section. In particular, look for carrots, corn, green peas, green beans, and broccoli.

To bring frozen veggies back to life, try steaming them on the stove top or cooking them in the microwave. Use as little water as possible, to preserve the nutrients. Prepared properly, frozen vegetables are just as nutritious as fresh.

Keep your grains whole. Whole grains are not only packed with vitamins and minerals, they're also loaded with fiber. And fiber makes you feel full, so you eat less—a big boost to weight loss.

One of the tastiest grains is rice—not the white instant rice, but brown and other varieties. Each has its own subtle flavor. Also shop for whole wheat pasta, barley, millet, bulgur, multigrain dinner rolls, and 12-grain breads.

Jazz up your meats. Worried that you can't survive on a smaller portion of meat? Intensify the flavor with herbs and spices, and you'll feel completely satisfied. You can do the same with your fish and poultry, too. At Canyon Ranch health resort in Tucson, culinary experts add crushed fresh herbs to 1 teaspoon of melted butter to create a richly flavored sauce for broiled fish. (While you should try to limit your intake of butter, which is pure saturated fat, using just a teaspoon wisely can make a big difference in your enjoyment of your meal.)

Keep in mind, too, that in terms of your sense of satisfaction, meal presentation is just as important as preparation. Foods should be as pleasing to your eyes as to your tastebuds. Three ounces of beef doesn't look paltry when it's sliced and arranged on your plate.

If you simply can't stop with 3 ounces, go ahead and help yourself to a larger serving. Then make your next meal vegetarian. To lose weight, you want to make dietary changes that you can live with.

Don't supersize your meals; undersize them instead. Always order a small.

"The portion sizes of typical servings have skyrocketed over the past several decades, leading many researchers to suggest that the huge portion sizes are a major contributing factor to the obesity epidemic, says Dr. Brill.

For example, a Coca-Cola in the early 1950s was just 6.5 ounces (and a mere 72 calories) whereas a Coca-Cola Classic "large" today—32 fluid ounces at McDonald's—contains a whopping 310 calories. Better to order a Coca-Cola Classic "child size" (at a reasonable 12 fluid ounces) for a much lower 110 calories. Even better, order an unsweetened iced tea, add some lemon juice and a packet of Splenda, and walk away with a refreshing drink for 0 calories and some extra nutrition (vitamin C from the lemon and disease-fighting polyphenols from the tea).

CHAPTER 21

THEY'RE LEAN AND LOVING IT

Sometimes it takes a good story to get us off our duffs and into walking. We like to hear that a person with whom we can identify worked out to lose weight and succeeded.

That's why we decided to collect several of our favorite "walking make-overs" and present them to you here. Between them, the four women whom we've profiled lost a total of 271 pounds. But it's not just their now-slim physiques that we find impressive. Each woman embodies the exhilaration of committing to a goal and achieving it. Success has changed them inside as well as outside.

58 POUNDS LIGHTER, HEALTHIER THAN EVER

At age 34, Lisa Baker seemed to be losing control of her health—and her life. She weighed 177 pounds, too much for her 5-foot-4 frame. She was on insulin to control her diabetes, a condition she'd had for 25 years, as well as medication for high blood pressure, an underactive thyroid, and sore feet. She took quinine for nighttime leg cramps and another drug for esophageal reflux. On top of all that, she developed a drinking problem.

Tired of feeling sick when she woke up in the morning, Lisa confided in a colleague, who referred her to a treatment program. As she began to feel better, she started walking, just around the block at first. "Three years earlier, I had managed to shed 30 pounds. But all of it came back, and then some," Lisa said.

Over time, her trips around the block extended to 4- to 5-mile daily excursions around several blocks, up hills, and over bridges. "Each day, I would try to walk just a little bit farther," she says. "Not so much that I felt uncomfortable, just enough to make a difference by the end of the week." Sometimes she'd listen to tapes of her favorite music, which helped to relieve stress. She also began lifting weights to build her upper-body strength.

Because she has diabetes, Lisa has very specific dietary guidelines to follow. But she taught herself to be more creative with her meals. "I used the American Diabetes Association diet as my guide," she explains. "For breakfast, I'd have bran cereal, half a pita, or a whole wheat bagel, plus a piece of fruit. Lunch might be turkey breast with low-fat cheese or salad greens or homemade lentil soup. On weekends when I had the grill out, I'd cook vegetables on it for a bit of variety."

Finally, Lisa was doing something good for herself, and it paid off handsomely. Within 2 years, her weight dropped to 119. Her nighttime leg cramps and reflux problems went away, and she no longer needed medication for blood pressure or painful feet. Her doctor reduced her insulin dosage from 38 units to 18. And she became alcohol free.

Lisa never imagined that walking could have such profound effects on her health. "I feel so much better, and I look better, too," she says. "That first walk around the block taught me an invaluable lesson: All things that seem insurmountable really do begin with a single step."

STAYING TRIM THROUGH TEAMWORK

As captain of the Buns and Roses walking team from Portland, Oregon, Jackie Lord is accustomed to rallying her teammates for competition. But it's her teammates who keep her motivated to walk and committed to fitness. She credits them with helping her to maintain an 80-pound weight loss for the past 4 years.

Jackie didn't always have a weight problem. In fact, as a high school student, she was a lean running machine.

At 5-foot-11 and a mere 125 pounds, she was fast enough to earn a spot in the Junior Olympics. But even then, despite her athletic prowess, she didn't pay much attention to eating right.

Years later, Jackie wed and began raising a family. The combination of a troubled marriage and a less-active lifestyle took a toll on her waistline. Eventually, she weighed 204 pounds. "When I turned 30, I joined Weight Watchers, where I lost 60 pounds," she says. "But as my marriage faltered, I got off track. I not only gained back the 60 pounds, but I added 60 more."

Jackie went back to Weight Watchers, but this time, she couldn't make it work. "I was having financial problems, and I just couldn't rationalize paying the fees," she explains. "So I decided to increase my activity level and watch my diet as best I could." On her own, she lost 80 pounds.

Suddenly, Jackie found herself facing a new dilemma. As thrilled as she was with her newly trim physique, she was terrified that all those pounds would come back. She knew she had to do something to stay motivated.

Jackie read several articles about walking and decided that it might help her trim and tone her body even more. At the time, her co-workers were looking for an organized activity that could help them shape up, too. So Jackie suggested that they form a team and enter the Portland to Coast Walk, a 127-mile walking relay event held every year in late August. They called themselves Buns and Roses and appointed Jackie captain.

In the relay, team members take turns walking 5- to 7-mile segments of the route. The entire event takes 20 to 24 hours to complete. "The first year we completed the relay, I cried for days afterward," Jackie says. "I couldn't believe that after years of abusing my body by gaining and losing weight, I was still able to accomplish such an athletic feat."

The experience proved emotional for another reason as well. "I remember coming down the promenade, about 300 yards from the finish line, when I spotted my daughter Kelly," Jackie says. "Kelly was our first-aid volunteer, but she's a star athlete in her own right, a state competitor in track and water polo. As I passed her, I could see that she was crying. She gave me a high five and told me that she was proud of me."

Kelly still calls her mom her hero, a title that Jackie treasures. It's one reason why she continues to enter Portland to Coast each year. Another is the camaraderie of her teammates. "We depend on each other for emotional support as well as physical motivation," Jackie explains. "In my case, the team keeps me committed to watching my weight and staying healthy. For others, the team has helped them to overcome weight problems, deal with divorces and the passing of loved ones, and confront emotional issues that deeply affect their lives."

Jackie, who's now married to a former member of the Buns and Roses volunteer support crew, says that her weight still fluctuates a bit. "But my doctor is thrilled with my cholesterol and sugar counts," she adds. "He says that I'm reducing my risk of diabetes, which runs in my family. And I feel as if I owe it all to Buns and Roses!"

SLIMMING HER BODY, HEALING HER MIND

Carol Fisher took up walking to slim down. Two years later, she was 35 pounds lighter. But that doesn't even compare to the weight of the stress that had been lifted from her shoulders, thanks to exercise.

"Back then, I was a newly single mom, working 60 to 70 hours per week just to provide the basic necessities for my three daughters," Carol recalls. "Eating was my main source of pleasure, a means of managing my stress. Only it didn't work."

Carol remembers sleeping poorly at night and being tired during the day. She felt like a failure, and it was crushing her spirit.

"My family had lost so much—our life, our home, our dreams," Carol explains. "There was no extra money for roller skates, bicycles, music lessons, or new clothes. I always dreamed of being a writer, but I no longer had the time, inspiration, or energy to write."

Carol hated the way she felt and looked. She knew that she had to do something, but what? Fitness centers and exercise equipment were out of the question—they were too costly. So were weight loss programs.

Carol mentioned her dilemma to a friend, who suggested that she start walking. After all, it was free—no expensive equipment or special clothing to buy, no diet pills to pop.

"That first morning, though, I would rather have faced a grizzly bear alone in the dark than dragged myself out of bed an hour early just to walk," Carol laughs. "As I headed out the door and down the sidewalk, I struggled with the idea that I had completely lost my sanity. Or that I might die from lack of sleep. Yet by the time I returned home, I hated to go back inside. It seemed like ages since I had breathed fresh air and heard the sounds of nature."

Getting up early never got easier for Carol, but that didn't stop her from becoming hooked on walking. Within several weeks, she realized that she was losing weight. "I no longer felt the need to eat so much," she says. "Even better, I was gaining energy and feeling less achy."

Walking also gave Carol the private time she needed to vent her grievances, clear her head, and pray for guidance. She began to think more clearly and to rediscover her life's dreams. Eventually, she decided that she wanted to go back to college. And she did.

Before Carol began walking, there was so much weighing her down, emotionally as well as physically. Today, she uses walking to keep her life on track. "If I feel my goals are slipping out of sight or becoming too hard to achieve, I take a walk," she says. "If I have issues that challenge and confuse me, I take a walk. When I need to talk or listen to God, I take a walk."

Yes, walking helped Carol to lose 35 pounds. But along the way, it also helped her to find herself.

MAKING WEIGHT LOSS PERSONAL

For Vicky Hager, losing and gaining weight was a way of life. She tried Weight Watchers and NutriSystem, once shedding more than 100 pounds. But the pounds were back within a few years.

By June 1995, Vicky's weight had crept to 264 pounds. "That's when I decided that I'd been fat long enough," she says. She was determined to slim down, and she'd do it on her own terms.

She combed through books and *Prevention* magazine, gathering information on weight loss. From that, she created her very own eating plan, breaking down her usual "three squares" into five mini-meals a day and counting grams of fat.

Once she got a handle on her eating habits, Vicky decided to add exercise to her weight loss program. She couldn't do much at first, but eventually, she was walking several miles a day.

"Near my home, there's a lake with a 2-mile path around it. My sister and I walked there at night," Vicky says. "At lunch, I'd do a 1-mile loop around town near my workplace." Once winter arrived, she moved her lunchtime workouts indoors, to the enclosed skywalks that crisscross downtown. In the evening, she'd stride on her treadmill or pedal her exercise bike.

"Eventually, I joined a fitness class that met on my lunch hour," Vicky says. "I never dreamed that I would join a fitness class at work!"

In May 1996, 11 months after launching her weight loss program, Vicky entered a 10-K with a partner. "We were the first to finish!" she says. "We were so proud."

The next month, Vicky traveled to Germany to visit her brother. "He was shocked by how good I looked and how fit I'd become," she smiles. "While I was there, we participated in four Volkswalks" (noncompetitive group walks).

Between her walking routine and her healthy eating habits, Vicky managed to lose 98 pounds in 1 year. At the time she shared her story, she wanted to lose 30 more. To help her reach her goal, she joined a weight loss support group. She also formed a group that gets together almost every day at lunch to walk.

"Right now, I walk 4 to 6 miles a day," Vicky says. "I feel great. I have lots of energy. And I do so many things that I never used to."

PART V

STRENGTH TRAINING FOR WALKERS

CHAPTER 22

A ROUTINE FOR THE ROAD

Do you want to add some oomph to your walking routine? Pick up your pace? Increase your mileage? Tackle steeper inclines?

The secret to walking faster, longer, and more energetically is a strong, limber body. That strength and flexibility can also help ward off pain in your shins and stiffness in your hips and lower back.

So how do you build such a powerful body? Easy: Just add some simple strength-training exercises to your workouts.

The following modest-but-mighty moves—recommended by walking coach Elaine Ward, founder and president of the North American Racewalking Foundation, and exercise physiologist Doug Garfield, EdD, developer of TrainS.M.A.R.T., a program for high-performance athletes—can make a huge difference in the effectiveness of your walking routine. The great thing about them is that they can be done on the go, without weights or other gadgets. The only "equipment" called for is the nearest tree or pole for balance.

You can incorporate these exercises into your workout any way you want. Do them all at once, or split them up between bouts of walking—walk for 10 minutes, do a set of an exercise, walk for 10 minutes, do a set of another exercise, and so on. If you close your eyes while you do the standing stretches, you will improve your balance as well.

To avoid muscle soreness, start with the smallest number of repetitions and work up gradually. Remember, too, that these numbers are only suggestions. If you need to start with fewer reps, that's fine. Allow your body to guide you.

Have fun—and get stronger fast.

PRIME YOUR SHINS FOR SPEED

If your shins scream, "Slow down!" whenever you make an effort to increase your pace, add either of the following exercises to your routine. You don't need to do both unless you have the time and the desire.

HEEL-TOE ROCK. With your weight balanced equally on both feet and your knees bent, gently rock back on your heels and pull your toes off the ground. Then with one smooth motion, rock forward and roll up onto your toes. Use all of your muscles to perform smooth, controlled movements. Do 12 to 15 repetitions, counting the entire heel-to-toe motion as one.

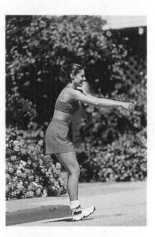

PAUSE WALK. Swing one leg forward as if to take a step. But before your heel hits the ground, pause with your foot about 3 inches off the ground and your toes pointed toward the sky. Slowly count to three, and as you do, continue pulling your toes back toward your shin. Repeat the pause with each step forward for 1 minute. Then walk normally for 1 minute. Repeat the entire cycle two more times.

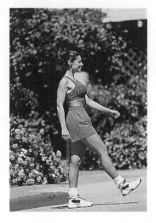

TONE YOUR HIPS FOR POWER

Strong, flexible hip flexor muscles add power and grace to your walk while helping you lengthen your stride. Try the following two exercises to limber up and increase your range of motion. They can also help alleviate any stiffness that you may notice after long periods of sitting.

FIGURE EIGHTS. Stand on one leg, holding on to a pole or a tree for support. With the opposite foot, draw a figure eight in the air, making the top loop in front of your body and the bottom loop behind your body. Gradually increase the size of the figure so that your hip rotates fully in front and back. Do 10 to 20 repetitions with each leg.

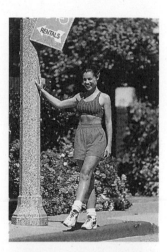

HIP STRETCH. This stretch is great for walkers as well as for anyone who has to sit most of the day. Stand tall, with your back straight. Step forward with your right leg, keeping your left foot on the ground. Make sure that your right knee is squarely over the center of your right foot, forming a 90-degree angle. Tilt your hips forward until you feel a mild stretch in your left hip. Keep your left heel flat. Hold for a slow count of five. Step back. Repeat two more times with your right leg forward, then switch legs to stretch your right hip.

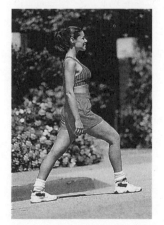

TIGHTEN YOUR TUMMY FOR ENDURANCE

Weak abdominal muscles contribute to poor posture and swayback, which can lead to back discomfort, especially on longer walks. These two crunches will help strengthen your stomach muscles and relieve back tension. And, even better, you don't need to lie down on wet grass to do them.

STANDING CRUNCH. Place your palms on the tops of your thighs. Round your back and contract your abdominal muscles. While crunching, slide your hands down your thighs to your knees, applying firm pressure along the way. This intensifies the contraction of your abdominal muscles. Relax. Do 12 to 15 repetitions.

TWISTING ABS. Place the palm of your right hand on top of your left thigh. Round your back and contract your abdominal muscles as you twist down and to the left. While crunching, apply firm pressure to your left thigh with your right hand to intensify the contraction of your abdominal muscles. Do 12 repetitions, then switch sides.

BUILD THIGHS TO CONQUER HILLS

If you walk on level ground most of the time, hills may seem especially challenging. That could be because your quadriceps, the muscles in the front of your thighs, aren't sufficiently developed. Practice these exercises every day, and you'll quickly turn mountains into molehills.

QUADS, PART 1. This is a controlled leg squat. Be sure to do it slowly so it feels challenging. Stand with your feet shoulder-width apart. Moving to a slow count of five, squat down as far as you comfortably can, but no farther than a 90-degree angle at your knees. Make sure that your knees are over but not past your toes and your back is straight. Then straighten up to a count of two. If you reach your arms overhead on your way up, you'll finish each squat by stretching your waist and rib cage. Work up to 15 to 20 repetitions. Always follow this exercise with Quads, Part 2.

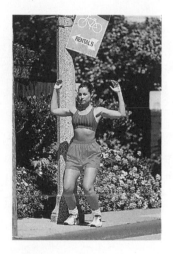

QUADS, PART 2. Stand with one foot on a curb, one in the street. Line up the toes of your street foot just below the instep of your curb foot. With your weight on your street foot, squat down to a count of two, then straighten up to a count of two. Again, don't bend your knees more than 90 degrees. You're using your whole body as a weight for your leg. Work up to 10 to 15 repetitions per side.

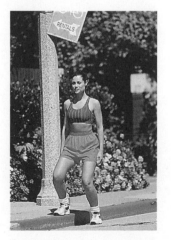

CHAPTER 23

MOVE SOME WEIGHT

We've already added some strength-training exercises to your workout in the previous chapter. Ready to take it a step further? Adding whole strength-training workouts to your overall exercise plan can dramatically increase your fitness. The American Diabetes Association recommends that people with diabetes do strength training several times a week to help build strong bones and muscles and make everyday chores such as carrying groceries easier. Plus, with more muscle, you burn more calories, even at rest. That will help if you're trying to shed some pounds.

Pick whichever of the following workouts most appeals to you and let's get moving . . . weights, that is.

STAND TALLER

Often when a person looks great, it's not their clothes or even their looks, it's their posture. Most of us tend toward muscular imbalance. Typically our chest and front shoulder muscles are stronger than our upper back and rear shoulder muscles. As a result, our chins jut out, our shoulders round, and our backs sway. Constant slumping increases the stress on the spine and joints and can lead to headaches, neck and shoulder tension, and lower-back pain. Strengthening and stretching the upper body will bring your muscles back into balance, improving your posture and making you look better in clothes. An added benefit: reduced neck and shoulder strain, which can decrease your risk of injury. Fortunately, good posture—like poor posture—is habit-forming. Do these few simple exercises four times a week to walk taller and stand straighter for life.

CHEST EXPANDER. Lie faceup with your legs bent and your feet flat on the floor. Bend your elbows and bring your forearms together over your chest, with your hands directly over your forehead and in a prayer position.

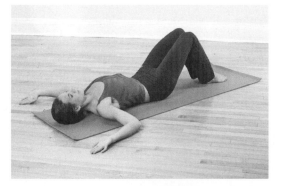

KEEPING your elbows bent at 90 degrees, lower your arms to the floor on either side of your head. You should feel your chest and shoulders opening and expanding. Hold for three breaths, then slowly lift your arms back to the starting position, feeling the stretch in your upper back and between your shoulder blades. Repeat 10 times.

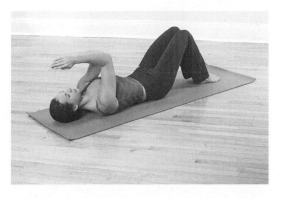

WALL ROLL-DOWN.

Stand with your back against a wall and your arms by your sides. Bring your heels together an inch or two from the wall; angle your toes out slightly.

CONTRACT your abs and relax your lower back, then roll down one vertebra at a time until your tailbone is all that touches the wall. Slowly reverse the move. Repeat three times.

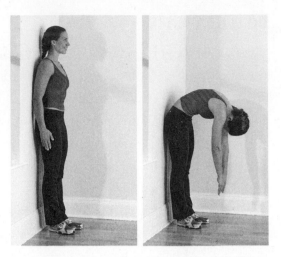

SHOULDER STRENGTHENER.

Stand with your feet hip-width apart, with your knees slightly bent, holding a 2- to 8-pound dumbbell in each hand. Keeping your back straight, bend forward 45 degrees at the hip. Let your arms hang down from your shoulders with your palms facing in.

SQUEEZE your shoulder blades together to raise the dumbbells 2 to 3 inches, then relax. Repeat 10 times.

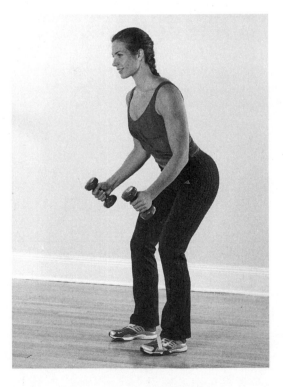

SCULPT SEXY ARMS

Do you feel your arms look flabbier these days? Age-related muscle loss does take a toll. But three simple strengthening moves are all you need to go sleeveless with confidence; you can see results in less than a month. Try this customizable triceps workout to build firm, shapely arms by spring—whatever your fitness level.

BALL PUSH-UP. First try this: Start on the floor in a push-up position, either on your knees or toes, with your hands beneath your shoulders and the ball under your left hand, with your fingers pointing forward. Inhale as you bend both of your elbows back, tucking them in to the sides, and lower your chest toward the floor. Exhale and push back to the starting position. Repeat. Halfway through the set, switch the ball to your right hand. (Bonus toning: chest, shoulders, and torso)

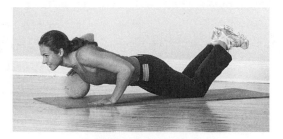

Make it easier: Skip the ball and place both of your hands on the floor under your shoulders.

Make it harder: Place both of your hands on the ball with your wrists facing and your fingers spread to the sides of the ball (not pictured).

Workout at a Glance

What you need: 3- to 5-pound dumbbells, a 9- to 10-inch-diameter ball (like a soccer ball, kickball, or medicine ball), and a sturdy chair.

How to do it: Do this routine 2 or 3 times a week on nonconsecutive days, completing 8 to 12 repetitions of each exercise. Begin with the First Try This move for each exercise. If it's too difficult, follow the Make It Easier variation. Not challenging enough? Try the Make It Harder option.

For quicker results: Do the entire workout twice through. As you get stronger and can breeze through 2 sets of 12 reps, progress to the next level or use a heavier weight.

CHAIR DIP. First try this: Sit on the edge of a chair with your feet flat and grasp the chair near your hips. Cross your right leg over your left, resting your ankle on your left thigh. Shift your hips off of the chair, supporting yourself on your hands and left foot. Make sure your left knee is over your ankle. Bend your elbows back, lowering your body until your arms are bent about 90 degrees, keeping your hips near the chair. Press into your palms, rising back to the starting position. Repeat. Halfway through the set, switch legs. (Bonus toning: shoulders and abs)

Make it easier: Keep both of your feet on the floor as you dip (not pictured).

Make it harder: Place your feet on the ball for an added balance challenge. Now lower, keeping your knees over your ankles (not pictured).

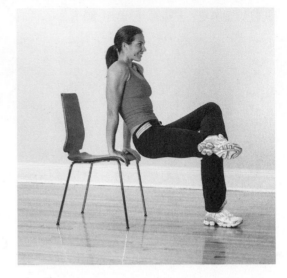

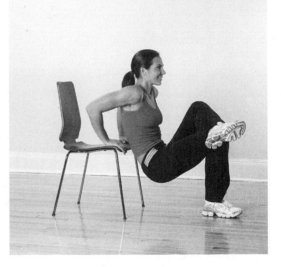

KICKBACK. First try this: Get down on all fours with your knees under your hips and your hands beneath your shoulders with your fingers pointing forward. Contract your abdominals and extend your right leg straight back, level with your torso. Grasp a dumbbell in your left hand, bending your arm to 90 degrees with your elbow at your side. Exhale and straighten your left arm, keeping your upper arm still and pressing the dumbbell back. Inhale and return to the starting position. After one set, switch sides. (Bonus toning: core and butt)

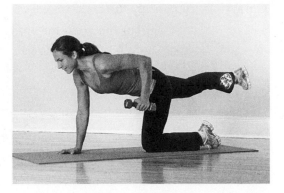

Make it easier: Start in the same tabletop position but keep both of your knees on the floor as you extend your arm behind you. After one set, switch arms and repeat (not pictured).

Make it harder: Stand with your weight on your right leg and a dumbbell in each hand. Hinge forward from your hips, raising your left leg behind until your torso and leg are parallel to the floor. Keeping your head in line with your spine, bend your arms 90 degrees with your elbows pulled in to your sides. Straighten and your bend arms. Halfway through the set, switch legs.

CINCH YOUR WAIST

In the hopes of creating a toned tummy, most people do sit-ups, which work the rectus abdominis, the long muscle between the ribs and the pelvis. But to really sculpt your abs, you must engage your entire torso. The three-dimensional moves in this routine zone in on your core by targeting your abs from every angle. They work the obliques on your sides, the transverse abdominis deep in your belly, and the muscles along your spine, in addition to the rectus abdominis.

Do two sets of 10 to 12 reps of each exercise, 5 days a week, and you'll show off a trimmer torso in just a month or two.

KNEE CIRCLES. Lie on your back with your arms resting at your sides. Raise your feet into the air and bring your knees over your rib cage.

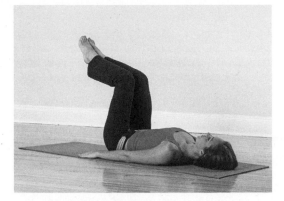

WITH your abs contracted and your belly pulled in toward your spine, slowly lower your knees to your side, then circle your knees away from you and around to the other side. Complete the circle by bringing your knees back to the starting position. Begin with small circles and increase the size for more of a challenge.

COMPLETE one set and repeat in the opposite direction.

DON'T arch your back

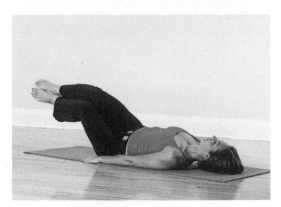

SIDE CHOP. Hold a 3- to 5-pound medicine ball or dumbbell and stand with your feet hip-width apart. Sit back into a half squat, contract your left obliques, and twist your torso to the left, bringing the ball to the outside of your left leg. Your knees should point forward and stay behind your toes.

As you stand back up, contract your right obliques and twist your torso to right, sweeping the ball up and across your body to the right. Follow the ball with your eyes until it's over your right shoulder. Return to the starting position and continue for one set. Switch sides and repeat.

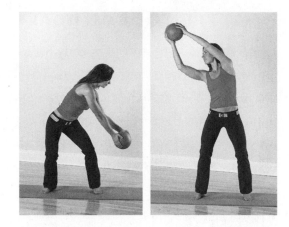

BACK EXTENSION. Kneel with your hands on the floor directly beneath your shoulders and your knees directly beneath your hips. Contract your abs and back muscles and simultaneously lift and straighten your left arm and right leg until they are in line with your torso. Hold for 3 seconds and lower. Complete one set; switch sides and repeat.

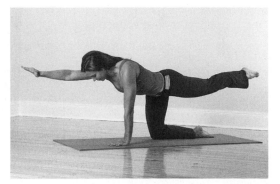

WHITTLE YOUR MIDDLE

If you think a bare midriff is only for teens, think again. You can show off your abs, too, with help from these exercises. They'll strengthen and tone the rectus abdominis, the muscle that stretches from your ribs to your hips, and the obliques, the muscles that run down the sides of your torso. Do two sets of 10 to 12 repetitions, with a 1-minute break in between. Aim for two or three workouts a week, resting a day between sessions, and you'll stand taller and look slimmer.

HIP LIFT. Lie on your back with your arms by your sides with your palms facing up. Raise your legs so they are straight up toward the ceiling and perpendicular to your torso.

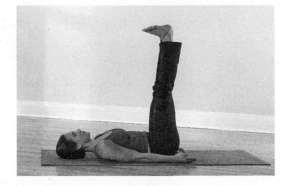

PULL your navel toward your spine and lift your hips a few inches off the floor, keeping your legs pointed straight up. Then slowly lower your hips back to the floor.

DON'T pull your legs toward your chest.

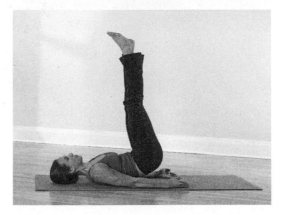

TORSO TWIST. Sit on the floor with your knees bent and feet flat, about hip-width apart. Extend your arms straight in front of you, and lace your fingers. Tighten your abdominal muscles and lean back about 45 degrees toward the floor.

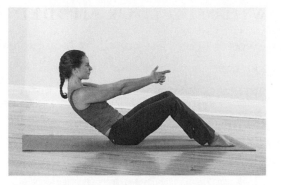

WITH your abs taut, rotate your torso toward the right as far as comfortably possible. Be sure to move your upper body (head, shoulders, arms, chest, and abs) in unison; don't lead with your arms. You should be looking in the same direction your hands are pointing throughout the move. Hold, then return to center and twist to the opposite side. That's one rep.

DON'T slump onto your lower back.

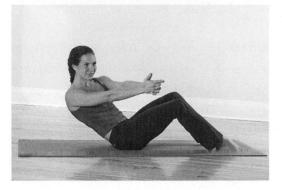

ENERGIZE AND FIRM YOUR LEGS

To counteract flab caused by too much sitting, simply lie back and put your feet up. Here are two moves for firming, lifting, and shaping your rear end and thighs that employ this principle. These lower-body toners use a stability ball and are done in a reclining position, so they're easier on your knees than squats. Keeping your legs elevated throughout each exercise also works your abs and increases circulation to energize your legs and reduce the risk of varicose veins. Do 2 or 3 sets of 10 to 12 reps of each move, 3 nonconsecutive days a week.

BRIDGE ROLL. Lie on your back with your arms at your sides and your heels on the ball. Lift your hips, lower back, and midback off of the floor.

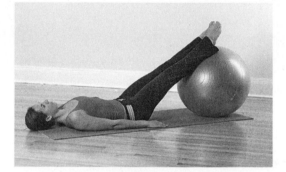

BEND your knees and roll the ball in toward your rear. Hold for a second, then extend your legs. Repeat. For more of a challenge, extend one leg toward the ceiling and roll the ball using only one leg at a time. (*Note:* This exercise is not recommended if you have back or neck problems.)

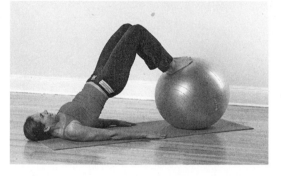

Quick Tip

Stability balls cost about $20 and are available online or wherever exercise equipment is sold.

CORKSCREW. Lie on your back, with your knees bent, and place the ball between your ankles. Squeeze the ball and extend your legs into the air.

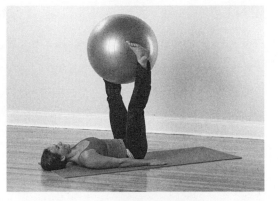

ROTATE your legs and the ball to the right, lowering your right leg. Hold for a second, then rotate to the left, raising your right leg and lowering your left. Hold and repeat. For more of a challenge, hold your legs at a 45-degree angle to the floor and rotate.

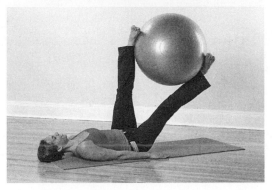

LEG STRETCH. Lie on your back with your legs straight and your heels on the ball. Raise your right leg off of the ball and grasp your calf or thigh, pulling your leg toward your head until you feel a gentle stretch. Hold for 20 seconds and release. Repeat with your left leg.

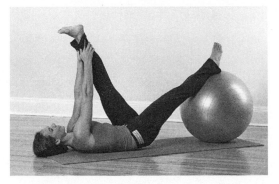

Quick Tip

For extra insurance against varicose veins and swelling, lie with legs propped up on the ball for 5 to 10 minutes a day.

CHAPTER 24

TRAINING FOR THE TRAILS

There's nothing like a hike to get you away from traffic, noise, and less-than-fresh air. But even dedicated city walkers might find themselves nursing sore feet, creaking knees, or an aching lower back after a day on the trail unless they do some prehike training.

This isn't to suggest that hiking is only for the superfit. On the contrary, anyone who's in reasonable shape can do it. But every activity uses certain muscles, and hiking uses different ones than walking.

To help prime your muscles for hiking, follow this training routine recommended by exercise physiologist Doug Garfield, EdD, developer of Train S.M.A.R.T., a program for high-performance athletes. His strategies can help you conquer any terrain and keep you from feeling overly sore the next day.

For the best results, practice these techniques for at least 2 weeks before you head out on the trail. By that time, you'll be not only stronger but also smarter about the demands of hiking and, therefore, less vulnerable to injury.

GET SET TO GO DOWNHILL

You may not think it, but descending a hill or mountain can be just as physically challenging as climbing up one. Each time your foot strikes the ground on your way down, it absorbs five times your body weight. On flat terrain, the impact is considerably less—just $1^1/_2$ times your body weight. You need to prepare your body for that extra stress.

"There is nothing like walking downhill to prepare you for hiking downhill," Dr. Garfield says. "It's the eccentric contractions (the lengthening of the leg muscles) that leave you stiff and sore the morning after your hike. To prepare your body for that, you need to find hills to walk down. No treadmill or stair-climbing machine can do it for you."

Try to incorporate walking downhill into the daily workouts leading up to your planned hike. Choose a slope that is paved or at least has an even surface. That way, you work your muscles properly and adequately without putting extra stress on your ankles and knees, which can occur when you're walking on a surface that's rutted, rough, gravel-covered, or just generally uneven.

DO A DRESS REHEARSAL

Another way to thwart posthike soreness is to wear your hiking shoes during your regular walking workout. They weigh more than your regular walking shoes, and they're designed differently, too. They'll take a little getting used to. "Consider this a dress rehearsal for your hike," Dr. Garfield advises. "You'll be much less likely to develop blisters or sore shins from the weight or friction of the boots."

Wearing your hiking boots before you go hiking may also help protect you against backache. "Many people experience lower-back pain after a day of hiking, and they think it's from carrying a pack," Dr. Garfield explains. "But often it's caused by the stress of wearing heavier shoes." The shoes give more momentum to your stride, making it longer. This change can tire out your lower back.

If you plan to carry a daypack when you go hiking, you ought to practice wearing it, too—during your walks around town or on your treadmill. "A pack changes your center of gravity and forces you to use your abdominal muscles more to maintain balance," Dr. Garfield explains. By working up to the approximate weight you'll be toting along on your hike, you'll be accustomed to the pack by the time you hit the trail.

SQUAT, THEN CLIMB ROCKS

For stepping from boulder to boulder and navigating loose accumulations of stone, you need stability in your lower

Buy the Right Boots

The type of shoes you wear is critical for people with diabetes, and hiking boots are no exception. Fortunately, hiking shoes today are a much better fit to the foot than shoes of 10 to 20 years ago. Plus, they're lighter and more breathable, which reduces the risk of infection or blistering, says Robert Katz, DPM, a podiatrist in Bradenton, Florida. Look for a shoe made out of materials that allow the foot to breathe while keeping moisture out, such as Gore-Tex.

body—your pelvis and hips as well as your knees and feet. This kind of stability comes courtesy of your torso muscles.

According to Dr. Garfield, one great way to toughen your trunk is to do squats. His technique: Pick up a soft exercise ball, the kind you might use in a swimming pool (not a Nerf ball, though). Make sure that it's soft enough to flatten out somewhat when you lean on it. Place it in the small of your back and lean against a wall. Slide down the wall into a squat, as though you are sitting down.

Go only as far as you feel comfortable, without straining. Ideally, your thighs should be parallel to the ground, but don't go any lower than that. Keep your knees aligned over your big toes and second toes. Then rise to the starting position. Gradually build up to 2 or 3 sets of 8 to 12 repetitions each.

This exercise helps stabilize your torso, pelvis, and hips by teaching you to equally support your weight in all directions as you roll the ball up and down the wall. It also helps strengthen your thighs, and it works fast.

CHAPTER 25

PAMPER YOURSELF WITH A PERSONAL TRAINER

Unless you use walking poles or an arm-pumping racewalking technique, your upper body probably isn't getting much of a workout when you walk. To give these muscles equal time, you need to add strength training to your exercise routine.

Strength training is an integral part of a total fitness program, even for the most dedicated walker. By increasing the strength of your arms, chest, shoulders, and back, you improve your posture and can carry boxes, bags, and other objects with ease. These changes enhance your overall sense of well-being.

Strength training can benefit your lower body, too. For example, if your regular walking route takes you over flat terrain, you're missing out on the buttock- and thigh-toning effects of climbing hills. Exercises that target these lower-body muscles can make a big difference in your physique. It may enhance your endurance while walking, too.

If you've never lifted weights before, or if you need extra motivation to stick with a strength-training program, consider signing on with a personal trainer. No class can compete with the one-on-one instruction that a personal trainer provides.

This fitness professional can teach you proper lifting technique, whether you're using free weights (dumbbells and barbells) or machines. You'll be amazed at how a slight variation in the way you hold a weight or position yourself on a machine can alter the effectiveness of an exercise. In fact, it can help protect you from injury.

HOW TO FIND A PERSONAL TRAINER

Before you start your search for a personal trainer, you need to decide whether you want to exercise at home or at a local gym or YMCA.

If you opt for the latter, then call the facility of your choice to inquire about the trainers it employs and the fees they charge. (Expect to pay between $30 and $40 an hour.) In general, gyms and Ys make sure that their employees have proper training and certification. They offer a variety of equipment, plus the motivation of seeing lots of people around you getting fit. Once you complete your training sessions, you can continue to use the facility for your workouts.

If you prefer to exercise at home, you need to buy some basic equipment. Initially, you may be able to get by with a few sets of hand weights. You'll likely pay more for a personal trainer, too— between $50 and $80 an hour. In return,

you have the convenience of a trainer who comes to you, at a time that works for you. This can be a real advantage if you have a busy schedule, as many people do. But when your training sessions are over, you'll have no one but yourself to keep you excited about your workouts. At a gym, sometimes just watching other people exercise helps boost your motivation to work hard and stick with your program.

Ideally, the trainer you choose should be certified by a reputable national fitness organization. The following are well known and, upon request, can provide listings of trainers by state.

- American Council on Exercise (ACE)— www.acefitness.org
- Aerobics and Fitness Association of America—www.afaa.com
- American College of Sports Medicine—www.acsm.org
- National Strength and Conditioning Association—www.nsca-lift.org

THE 10 BIGGEST FITNESS BLUNDERS

ACE polled its trainers to find out the most common mistakes people make when exercising. At the very least, these errors undermine the effectiveness of a workout. At worst, they may lead to strain, pain, and injury.

1. Not stretching enough: Whether you're exercising aerobically or lifting weights, warm up first, then stretch.
2. Lifting too much weight: Increase your weight gradually, and you'll avoid setting yourself up for pain.
3. Not warming up before an aerobic activity: Don't set the treadmill to your fastest pace as soon as you step on. Gradually increase your speed.
4. Forgetting to cool down: Before you head for the showers, cool down by doing some light activity, such as walking slowly. Then stretch your muscles to improve their flexibility. You're actually getting them ready for your next workout.
5. Exercising too hard: If you've skipped several workouts, don't try to make up for lost time in one session. You're only setting yourself up for soreness and possible injury.
6. Drying up: Drink lots of water before, during, and after your workout.
7. Leaning on the stairclimber rails: Yes, you can burn more calories by exercising on a stairclimbing machine than by walking. But if you lean on the handrails during your workout, you're just defeating the purpose.
8. Wimping out: While you don't want to push yourself too hard, especially if you're just starting an exercise program, you need to work intensively enough to get results. It's a fine balance—one that's much easier to maintain with the guidance of a personal trainer.
9. Jerking the weight: In strength training, you control the weight. Make your moves smooth. If you jerk when you lift, you need a lighter weight.
10. Pigging out: If you're at the gym for less than 2 hours, you don't need to supplement your meals with sports drinks and energy bars. A healthy, balanced eating plan and plenty of water will cover your nutritional bases.

PART VI

THE SPIRIT IN WALKING

CHAPTER 26

SLOW DOWN TO
THE SPEED OF WALKING

If you're like most people, you've taken up walking to improve yourself physically, perhaps by slimming down or getting fit. But there's another side to walking, one that supports your emotional and spiritual being, that lets you escape some of the craziness of 21st-century living.

These days, our lives are set at an incredibly frantic pace. We have so much on our plates that we fear we'll never get everything done. And we wonder when we'll find time to do those things that bring us pleasure and joy.

Even when the world seems to be spinning out of control, walking can restore your sense of inner peace. It gives you a chance to slow down, to relax, to appreciate yourself and your life. Time seems to expand, creating a sense of spaciousness in the present moment.

Even if your job is wonderful, your family is healthy and happy, and your future seems bright, you can lose touch with the deepest part of yourself unless you slow down enough to breathe deeply, to still your thoughts, to observe the natural world with a sense of wonder. In this regard, walking can help you reset your internal clock and dispel your sense of urgency. After all, it isn't intended to get you someplace in a super-hurry—unless you're an elite racewalker. By its very nature, it encourages you to breathe more deeply, draining away tension and instilling a sense of calm and contentment.

PLAN A WALKING RETREAT

You can use walking as a sort of mini-retreat. You don't have to go away for a week or even a weekend, unless you want to, of course. Just set aside 1 day for a 3- to 8-hour exploration on foot—far from the demands of work, home, and family.

First, choose a date on your calendar and mark it as your "retreat day." Then discuss your plans with anyone who might be affected by your being unavailable. You want this day to be yours, for your personal walking adventure. (You can invite a friend or family member to join you if you want. But we suggest that you make all the plans so that they suit *you*.)

Next, identify a place that you want to explore on foot. If you enjoy being out in nature, call the local parks and recreation department to request maps of that area. If you love looking at homes and gardens, think of a neighborhood that you'd like to see up close. Try to choose a location that's no more than 15 minutes from your home. You want to spend your time walking, not driv-

ing. If you never have to get in your car, all the better.

Tailor the length of your route to your personal limits. You're walking at a leisurely pace, so you can go longer and farther. If you normally walk 2 miles a day, go for 4 to 6 miles. If you usually walk 4 miles, try to go 8 to 10. If you're a beginner, stay under 4 miles.

The night before your excursion, pack yourself a lunch, maybe a sandwich on whole grain bread, plus fresh fruits and veggies. Make sure that you have a water bottle, too. Put them in a backpack, along with a notepad and pencil in case you want to do some journaling. Other items you may want to carry along include any maps you need; pocket guides for identifying wildflowers, trees, and birds; a magnifying glass for checking out the intricacies of plants; a couple of premoistened hand wipes; and some plastic bags for any garbage you have.

Make sure your favorite walking socks are clean. Pick out a pair of shorts or pants that you can walk in comfortably for hours as well as a cozy jacket if the weather is cool. If it's warm, wear a hat or visor. And don't forget your sunglasses—not only to shade your eyes but also to give you a sense of privacy while you walk.

EXPLORE THE WORLD . . . AND YOUR SOUL

On the day of your journey, plan to get up early, so you can spend a few minutes relaxing and stretching. Stretching is something few people make time for, but it yields great rewards. It leaves you feeling lighter, more flexible, less achy. It makes your walk more refreshing, since you've worked out some of the kinks before you hit the road. So indulge yourself in a long, soothing stretching session. If you have a favorite yoga video, pop that in and follow along.

If you have a favorite book of poetry, read from it before you leave home. The sensuous, intuitive language of poetry may put you in a completely different frame of mind than the articles in the morning paper. Afterward, eat a healthy breakfast and drink plenty of water. Then pick up your backpack and head out.

Remember, this is a retreat, not a race. Training for a 5-K or a 10-K is a whole other objective. This is to refresh your spirit, to get in sync with your soul and your surroundings. Stand tall while you walk; it makes you feel better about yourself and the world around you. Stop whenever you want to eat a midmorning snack or your lunch. Soak up the sun. Stretch again. Savor the moment.

CHAPTER 27

SKY WALKING:
A NEW VIEW OF THE WORLD

So you've already done your walking for the day. Quick—without taking your eyes off this page—try to remember what the sky looked like while you were outside. What was its color? Were there any clouds? What did they look like? Were they moving slowly or quickly?

If you're like most people, you probably can't give a detailed description of the sky's appearance, even though you were surrounded by it, says Jack Borden, founder of For Spacious Skies, a nonprofit organization based in Lexington, Massachusetts. And that's too bad. Because by focusing your eyes on the sky and really studying it, you can boost the de-stressing effects of your walks.

SEEKING HELP FROM ABOVE

Ralph Waldo Emerson, a 19th-century poet and an avid walker, once described the sky as "the daily bread of the eyes." Borden got a monumental mouthful of it one day 10 years ago, as he rested in a meadow after a long hike. "I looked up, and for the first time in my life, I saw the sky," he recalls.

Realizing what he had been missing, he quit his job as a television broadcaster and founded For Spacious Skies, which is devoted to increasing people's awareness of the sky. Some of what Borden has learned from looking up could add a new dimension to your walking program—and to other parts of your life as well.

LOOKING UP, LOOKING IN

Psychological research suggests that the rewards of really seeing the sky may be greater than just a pleasant feeling from having taken in a nice view. Specifically, sky gazing may sap stress by helping you put your emotions in perspective. As Borden explains, "When you realize that everyone is *in* the sky instead of *under* it, as many people perceive themselves, you get a stronger sense of connectedness."

Ecopsychologist Sarah Conn, PhD, agrees that walkers have much to gain by tuning in to the sky. (Ecopsychology is a relatively new field of study in emotional and mental health. It's based on the philosophy that people are connected to more than just the human world and are profoundly influenced by that connection.) According to Dr. Conn, awareness of the sky can help anyone under stress experience their situations in a larger context. They may be able to take that feeling of space outside themselves and somehow translate it to a feeling of spaciousness within themselves.

"In addition, watching the sky and the changes that steadily occur in it can give people a sense that their own feelings move the same way," Dr. Conn says. "Stormy or gentle, feelings all come and go. But above the clouds, the sky is always there, always blue."

GETTING THERE FROM HERE

For some people, a good look up to the heavens is all they need to experience the sky's stress-reducing powers. Others might get better results by using one of these two approaches.

Turn outward. Dr. Conn reminds you to "stay out of your head" when you walk. "One Native American phrase for insanity translates as 'talking, talking, talking, inside your head,'" she notes. "When people keep up this incessant internal chatter, they don't get relief on their walks. I remind them to stop, look, listen, smell, and touch the world around them."

When you're out walking, use all your senses. Taste the air, feel the wind, touch a tree. Try to walk in the same place often, and pay careful attention to the changes that occur from one visit to the next. This includes the changes that take place overhead in the sky. "All this creates a wonderful sense of connectedness and comfort," Dr. Conn says. "The natural world is a place where you don't have to perform. You can act or feel however you want, and the sky is just there."

By walking with awareness of the natural world—of the ground beneath your feet, of the scents, sounds, and smells—you develop a very real protection against stress, according to Dr. Conn. "Stress can move through you more quickly and with greater ease," she explains.

Reframe what you see. It's easy to feel distressed or overwhelmed when some part of your life's landscape is in disarray. Borden recommends an exercise from Apache culture to help you see that any ugliness is only a small corner of your personal picture.

As an example, imagine that you're walking near your town's dump, and you feel overwhelmed by its ugliness. Look out toward the horizon and try to see as much of the landscape as you can, horizontally and vertically. Get the biggest picture that you can without focusing on any one object in particular.

Pretend that your eye is a camera lens. Look closely at the dump through that lens. Then turn the lens toward the sky. As you take in the sky's beauty, you become unaware of the dump. Tilt the lens again until you see only the dump. Then shift back to the big picture, combining the sky and the dump. This is a truer picture of reality—80 percent beauty, 20 percent ugly. You'll feel not only less anxious about the ugliness but also empowered to do something about it if you want to.

Of course, you don't have to limit your awareness of the sky to your walks. Try turning off the television one evening and taking your family outside for some stargazing. Or spend a lazy summer day lying faceup on the lawn, letting the sky sap away your daily stresses. Even these simple acts can be truly potent tools for reframing your thoughts about life.

CHAPTER 28

LABYRINTH WALKING: A PATH TO INNER PEACE

Going around in circles has never been considered a good thing. It means that you're getting nothing accomplished on a certain project or task.

When you walk a labyrinth, you go around in circles. The difference is, you actually get somewhere. In fact, you follow a path to remarkable stress reduction and relaxation.

Labyrinths are cropping up in parks and on parking lots, in public places and on private property. These intricate courses with ancient roots continue to grow in popularity, as people discover their power to calm the mind and soothe the body. To experience their appeal for yourself, all you have to do is walk between the lines.

Most people think of a labyrinth as a maze from which there is seemingly no escape. But the type of labyrinth we're talking about is two-dimensional, with no walls to obstruct your vision. It's also unicursal, which means it has a single, winding path that leads to a central point. Follow the path to get to the center, then follow it back to the starting point. No directions, no decisions, and no getting lost.

A maze, on the other hand, has many paths (it's multicursal), and most of them lead to dead ends. Walking a maze is a challenge that can require stamina. Walking a labyrinth requires only that you persist in your journey.

FIND YOUR WAY WITHIN

As with so many things in life, what you get out of a labyrinth depends a great deal on what you put into it, says Robert Ferre, director of Labyrinth Enterprises and author of *The Labyrinth Revival.* "You can skip through the winding paths with childlike abandon, or you can walk solemnly and introspectively."

Many say that walking a labyrinth calms the body and mind by providing a space that guides a person's focus inward. The rhythmic action of walking can reduce the nervous energy that prevents some people from reaping the benefits of other relaxation techniques. And when you walk a labyrinth, the effortlessness of following the winding path deepens your breathing and helps to release built-up tension.

Some people find inspiration or solve problems on the labyrinth path. Others walk to help them focus at the beginning of the day. Of course, you can experience these benefits on any path. But labyrinth enthusiasts, including art therapist Annette Reynolds, RN, feel that the intricate courses offer a special format for "going within."

"I've attended classes in therapeutic touch [which some call the *laying on of hands*]," Reynolds says. "A friend of mine described walking a labyrinth as the laying on of feet. That's how I see it. I've even built one in my garden for my personal use."

A UNIFYING FORCE

Communities are using labyrinths to foster unity by inviting everyone to "walk the path together," a symbolic act of cooperation.

For example, as part of a First Night (New Year's Eve) celebration in St. Peters-

---

Labyrinth Locating

To find a labyrinth in your area, or to find out more about labyrinths in general, visit the Web site of the Labyrinth Society, www.labyrinthsociety.org, or call toll-free at 877-446-4520. The Web site offers a worldwide labyrinth locator and a virtual labyrinth walk that you can enjoy from your computer.

Sacred Strolls

Any discussion of labyrinth walking would be incomplete without mention of the role of churches in reviving the ancient practice. Since the publication of *Walking a Sacred Path* by the Reverend Dr. Lauren Artress, a licensed therapist and canon for special ministries at Grace Cathedral in San Francisco, labyrinths have been cropping up at churches around the country.

Historically, pilgrims walked labyrinth paths as a symbolic journey to Jerusalem, following the footsteps of Jesus. Today, labyrinths serve as a metaphor for the spiritual journey through life, as a source of solace and spiritual introspection, as a setting for religious ceremonies, and as a tool for everyday focusing.

Dr. Artress describes walking the labyrinth as a form of prayer called *body prayer.* "The labyrinth reintroduces us to the experience of walking a clearly defined path," she explains. "It reminds us that there is a process that brings us to unity, to the center of our beings. In the simple act of walking, the soul finds peace."

burg, Florida, organizers created a labyrinth on the site of a demolished downtown building. Their goal was to address racial discord and promote community involvement. "As people walked toward the center of the labyrinth, they were to think about what they would do to help heal the city," explains G. David Ellis, the course designer. "When they got to the center, they tied ribbons to a pole as a symbol of commitment. Then as they walked back, they were to contemplate how to make their pledges a reality."

The event was an enormous success. The labyrinth was packed all evening, and by the time it closed, more than 3,000 ribbons adorned the center pole. It was community art in its highest form.

STAY THE COURSE

If you're a newcomer to labyrinth walking, you may not be sure what to expect from the experience. Ferre advises that you "set aside any preconceived notions or skepticism and be open to whatever happens." And be sure to follow these basic rules of labyrinth etiquette.

1. Begin only at the entry point.

2. Time your start so that people walking ahead of you don't feel rushed or crowded.

3. Walk on the path, not on the lines or markers.

4. Set your own pace.

5. Pass others if necessary, and allow others to do likewise.

6. If possible, sit quietly at the center of the labyrinth before heading back. (At large events, you may be asked to keep moving, since the course can become crowded.)

7. Honor specific requests—for silence, for example.

Create Your Own Labyrinth

Labyrinths have various configurations. They can be as simple as a sand drawing or as elaborate as an inlaid tile floor.

The classic and simple seven-circuit labyrinth has been in existence for more than 4,000 years. Its history extends to a diverse array of cultures, including Native American, Scandinavian, and Indian. Its circular paths have been captured in ancient cave paintings and carved into the turf of a grassy knoll in England. The paths are easy to replicate.

A second, more complex type of labyrinth developed during the Middle Ages. It's found primarily in churches, with the most famous example being the inlaid floor design of Chartres Cathedral in France. These labyrinths are being copied onto canvases and circulated from community to community for retreats and celebrations.

If you're really into labyrinth walking, you can build a course in your own backyard. It doesn't have to be as elaborate as the ones described above. The Labyrinth Society offers instructions on how to build a classic seven-circuit labyrinth on its Web site, www.labyrinthsociety.org. Also, Labyrinth Enterprises, formerly known as the St. Louis Labyrinth Project, sells books and instructions for making a Chartres pattern labyrinth and a classic seven-circuit labyrinth on its Web site, www.labyrinth-enterprises.com.

CHAPTER 29

WELCOME TO YOUR CREATIVE ZONE

On any given day, you probably face at least one problem or task that demands a bit of creative thinking on your part. Here's an easy way to get those creative juices flowing: Just put one foot in front of the other.

That's right. Research has shown that in addition to its myriad health benefits, walking can actually enhance creativity. In one study, all 63 participants reported a significant increase in the flow of ideas after just 25 minutes of aerobic activity. That's a benefit worth striding for.

Want to brainstorm money-saving initiatives for your boss? Plan a birthday party for your spouse? Redesign your kitchen? Whatever the situation, if it requires brainpower, try foot power.

LET YOUR MIND ROAM FREE

What is it about moving your arms and legs that seems to turbocharge your brain cells? Scientists theorize that exercise causes the brain to enter a state of relaxation. In this looser mind-set, thoughts that would normally be stored in separate compartments instead become blended together. The result is a delicious stew of new ideas.

Creativity coach Julia Cameron, author of *The Artist's Way*, prescribes a daily walk as a potent source of inspiration. "Walking feeds us, image by image. It's one of the most powerful creative tools I know," she says. "With the constant inflow of new images, walking gives us new thoughts that nourish us. It replenishes our overtapped creative well and gives us a sense of . . . well, wellness."

When you're out walking—away from ringing telephones, pressing deadlines, and other nagging responsibilities—you feel free to let your imagination play. The busy owner of one New York City public relations firm couldn't agree more. "I run a company, and I have a family," the woman says. "When I'm walking, no one is making demands on me. It's amazing what your mind can do when it's not being pushed and prodded in six different directions."

Dedicated walkers report that they enjoy a wide variety of mind-metamorphosing benefits. Creativity, after all, takes countless forms—from penning prose to resolving sticky situations, from communing with nature to connecting with your innermost spirit.

WALKING TO WORK SMARTER

For many people in "creative" professions, walking is a direct path to doing better work. "During one walk, I came up with an entire section of a speech that I was to give at an awards luncheon,"

says a senior vice president of Minkus and Dunne Communications, a Chicago-based public relations firm.

Paul Levinson, PhD, professor and chair of the department of communication and media studies at Fordham University in New York City, is the author of seven books, 30 science fiction stories, and 100-plus scholarly articles. He has done most of his writing since 1993, the year he started walking. He says that's no coincidence.

"Walking opens my mind to ideas that have been nesting in there for years," Dr. Levinson observes. "It took me at least 5 years to write my 1988 book, *Mind at Large*. I completed my latest book, *The Soft Edge*, in 5 months. There's no doubt that walking has made my writing more creative."

PROBLEM SOLVING, STEP BY STEP

Walking can do much more than enhance job performance. For many people, it leads to the discovery of a solution to some professional or personal challenge.

"It doesn't always happen instantly, but over time, you go from worrying about problems to finding ways to address them," Cameron says. "In some cases, the solutions may seem crazy at first. But the more you think about them, the smarter they become."

That busy New York City PR executive uses her frequent walks to untangle all manner of perplexing knots, from reorganizing her office staff to deciding what to feed her family for dinner. "You've heard about how your mind can work on problems while you're sleeping? I think the process is analogous to that," she says. "Your mind is working on your problem while you're walking, even if you're not consciously aware of it."

MAKE WALKING A CREATIVE VENTURE

You can't force creativity. But you can give it a gentle nudge by walking. Experts offer these strategies to help you use walking to stimulate your creative processes.

Exercise every day. Cameron prescribes a 20-minute walk 6 days a week, plus an hour-long walk once a week. "The idea is to stretch both your legs and your creative territory," she says.

Find the right time. Try to do your walking when you can disengage yourself from schedules and structures. "The human mind generally can't switch off old business like a light, so you should walk at a time when you can let go," advises James A. Swan, PhD, an environmental psychologist in Mill Valley, California, and author of *Nature as Teacher and Healer.*

Dr. Levinson agrees, adding that his best creativity-generating walks occur between 10:00 and 11:00 at night. "Afterward, I produce about 2 hours' worth of good writing," he says.

Find the right place. According to Cameron, where you do your walking doesn't matter all that much, as long as it's outside in a place in which you feel safe and comfortable. (While treadmills provide exercise, they don't provide the "image flow" required for creativity.) Head out on your own and see where it leads you.

Attend to your mind. While you walk, focus on what you see, hear, and feel, Dr. Swan suggests. At first, you may be restless or feel overwhelmed by the plethora of images that flood your mind. But eventually, your mind will get in sync with the beauty and stimulation of your environment. Over time, you'll find yourself having larger, simpler, and unique creative insights. Step by step, you'll learn to put greater trust in your own ideas. "You'll know they're right because they feel right," he says.

CHAPTER 30

RECONNECT WITH
THE NATURAL WORLD

In the 21st century hustle and bustle, it's not uncommon for people to go from house to car to work and back again without spending more than a few minutes outside. We live our lives in air-conditioned boxes, separated from nature by wood, stone, and steel.

Yet given the time and freedom to step outside of our boxes, we realize how nature can strengthen and sustain us. Feel the warm sun on your face, hear the wind in the trees, and smell the fresh air. Reconnect with nature!

One study found that walking in nature has even more health benefits than most of us imagined. In the study, researchers at the University of Michigan School of Nursing in Ann Arbor noticed that of 32 women being treated for localized breast cancer, those who received a 20- to 30-minute "dose" of nature-based activity every week showed improvement in their ability to think clearly, to set goals, and to start a task and follow through. The researchers identified other benefits, too, including a resurgence in energy and optimism that encouraged the women to take on new tasks, such as volunteer work, or to learn new skills.

None of this will surprise experts in ecopsychology, a field of study that views people as profoundly affected by the natural world. Michael J. Cohen, EdD, author of *Reconnecting with Nature*, offers the following exercises to help you reconnect with nature and, in doing so, to connect more deeply with yourself. You can transform your walks into moving meditations that calm, refresh, and revitalize you.

EXERCISES FOR THE SENSES

These exercises are intended to awaken or sharpen senses that you probably haven't paid much attention to. By using these senses to explore the natural world, you come to realize that you're part of nature, not apart from it. According to Dr. Cohen, this realization helps people learn to make healthier decisions, both for themselves and for their environments.

Ultimately, the goal of the exercises is to help you understand the relationship between your psychological health, your sense of well-being, and the health of the environment around you. You make this critical connection by becoming aware of all the sensory interactions that exist within the natural world.

SAY HELLO TO MOTHER NATURE

The value of the exercises lies solely in your experience of them. If you just read them, they may seem, quite simply, silly. But if you do them and have fun with them, you may find a whole new pleasure and energy in walking outdoors.

Plan to do no more than one exercise a day. "Trying to do all of them in one day dilutes your experience," Dr. Cohen says. "You probably won't sense as much."

If you find that you're not attracted to a particular exercise, put it off for another day or skip it completely. If you find that you don't trust your own reactions at times when doing the exercises, sharing your feelings or insights with a friend or a group really helps.

Keep in mind, though, that there are no right or wrong results. Just enjoy yourself!

Explore without your eyes. This is a great technique for awakening your senses before you start walking. Find a spot in your yard or in some natural area where you can stand quietly with your eyes closed. (If it's outside your yard, make sure that it's a place where you feel completely safe.) If you're comfortable doing so, walk around slowly, keeping your eyes closed. Become aware of the input you're receiving from your other senses now that your dominant sense, your vision, is "turned off."

Listen, smell, and—if the area is free of potentially harmful plants (such as rose bushes and poison ivy)—touch as you explore your surroundings. Notice as many sensations as you can. Pay attention to your sense of the ground underfoot, your sense of balance, and your sense of direction based on the sun or the wind. Notice whether you can feel the presence of trees or rocks around you without touching them. Occasionally open your eyes for just a second and notice how your environment looks. Many people report a heightened awareness of color and shape.

See with your hands. Before you begin walking, go outside and pick up five or six pebbles or small stones of similar shape and size. Mark one with a felt marker or pen. Put the rest in your pocket.

Hold the marked stone in your hand as you walk, learning to recognize it by touch. After 5 to 10 minutes, drop the stone into your pocket with the others and mix them up. Then without actually looking in your pocket, reach in and see if you can pick out the marked stone. Repeat the activity with new stones, or just mark a different stone. It's remarkable how different each stone really feels, even though they all look the same.

Connect with your breath. For this exercise, all you do is think about breathing. Remember that plants release the oxygen that you breathe into your lungs; in return, you breathe out the carbon dioxide that plants take in.

In your mind's eye, follow your breath as you exhale. Imagine that you can see the carbon dioxide molecules leaving your nose or mouth and flowing into the leaves of the plants nearest you as you walk. At the same time, envision yourself inhaling the oxygen that the plants give off. Take a moment to note how your visualization of this very natural process affects your sense of the world around you.

Acknowledge your appreciation. Think of the wonderful feeling that you get when you say thank-you to someone who has given you a gift or a compliment. When you see a beautiful tree and you stop for a moment to experience your appreciation of its beauty, you're sending a mental thank-you to that tree. Can the tree sense your gratitude? Who knows. But try this exercise and notice how it affects your perception of the world around you.

First, suspend any preconceived notions of what's pleasing or attractive. You may be drawn to a certain color, a particular smell, a certain view, or something else. As you become aware of the object or the environment, take a moment to appreciate that it has made you feel good. Dr. Cohen suggests that you even mentally thank whatever has attracted you.

At the end of your walk, write your experience in a logbook. Finish this statement: "I am a person who appreciates and feels supported by . . . " Fill in the blank with what you felt attracted to.

Happy Trails to You

Where did your search for nature lead you? Likely to one of the many trails running through local, state, and national parks.

Of course, trails don't just happen. They must be built and maintained, and that costs money. A portion of our local, state, and federal tax dollars are earmarked for this purpose. But this financial support can quickly disappear—unless we let our government officials know that the trails are important to us.

That is why the American Hiking Society sponsors National Trails Day, held the first Saturday of every June to draw attention to and celebrate America's walking, hiking, and biking trails. Hundreds of thousands of people take part in more than 1,000 activities in venues across the country. By joining them, you not only get your weekly dose of nature but also send a message to your government officials that you care about and enjoy having access to trails.

Through this annual event, the American Hiking Society is working toward two goals: to give everyone in the United States trail access within 15 minutes of home and to develop a trail network that could take us wherever we wanted to go, from sidewalk to backwoods. A grand vision? Of course! But one that's worth walking toward, considering its benefits.

For more information about National Trails Day events in your area, visit the American Hiking Society's Web site, www.americanhiking.org, or call 301-565-6704.

CHAPTER 31

ON FOOT AND ON FAITH: THE STORY OF PEACE PILGRIM

She didn't wear high-tech walking shoes, just plain canvas sneakers. She didn't sport a jacket or hat with a famous logo, just a simple navy blue tunic and pants. No organization sponsored her. No one followed her with a van to pick her up when she grew tired or when the weather turned foul. She traveled alone, on foot and on faith, with a singular purpose: to share her prescription for worldwide harmony. "Overcome evil with good, falsehood with truth, and hatred with love. This is the way to peace," she told anyone who stopped to ask.

In the past century and a half, countless people have walked countless miles on countless missions. Many of these walkers deserve recognition for their feats. One very special walker was a blue-eyed, slightly wizened marvel who spent almost three decades trekking across the United States on foot.

Her name was Mildred Norman Ryder, but she became known simply as Peace Pilgrim. The name captured her essence: She was a woman on a 25,000-mile walking pilgrimage for peace.

In the 1950s, long before T-shirts became billboards for personal politics, Peace Pilgrim realized that sewing a few words to her tunic—"Walking Coast to Coast for Peace"—would be an effective way to share her message with others.

Peace Pilgrim was a phenomenal walker, in every sense of the word. She covered an astonishing number of miles in her lifetime, many more than the 25,000 she originally set out to do. Even more impressive, she accumulated most of that mileage *after* her 50th birthday. She was vital, energetic, and at peace with herself. She was amazing.

WALKING TOWARD A VISION

Walking played an integral part in the "creation" of Peace Pilgrim. During what she described as her 15-year preparation period, Peace—then known simply as Mildred—spent time every day walking and drawing inspiration from nature. She said that she received insights on those daily walks, and she worked to incorporate those insights into her daily life. She encouraged others to do the same. "From the beauties of nature, you get your inspiration," she once said. "From the silent receptiveness, you get your meditation. From the walking, you get not only exercise but deep breathing—all in one lovely experience."

In 1952, a year before her first sojourn as Peace Pilgrim, Mildred walked the entire Appalachian Trail, from Maine to Georgia, a distance of more than 2,000 miles. It taught her the necessity of traveling light. "I lived out-of-doors completely, supplied with only one pair of slacks and shorts, one blouse and sweater, a lightweight blanket, and two double plastic sheets into which I sometimes stuffed leaves," she said. "I was not completely dry and warm, but I enjoyed it thoroughly!"

Toward the end of her Appalachian expedition, after walking all night, Mildred had a vision of her first pilgrimage across the country. That's when Peace Pilgrim was born.

SPREADING A MESSAGE OF PEACE

Peace Pilgrim's monumental trek across the United States began in 1953 at the Tournament of Roses Parade in Pasadena, California. There she handed out leaflets and gathered signatures for a Peace Petition, which she delivered to the United Nations after walking coast to coast. Until her death in 1981, she crisscrossed the country seven times on foot, stopping to talk with anyone intrigued by the message emblazoned on her tunic.

Like some spiritual Johnny Appleseed, Peace Pilgrim sowed the seeds of her mission through one-on-one conversations, college lectures, church services, radio programs, and TV interviews. She covered, as she liked to say, "the whole peace picture—peace among nations, peace among groups, peace among people, and, most important, inner peace." It wasn't a new message; she openly acknowledged that. But it was a message that she felt America needed to hear.

Day in and day out, regardless of the season, Peace Pilgrim wore the same outfit. She washed her garments in restrooms, then allowed them to air-dry on her body. Changes in the temperature didn't slow her down; she said that her body had learned to quickly adjust to weather conditions. She ate only when she was offered food and slept wherever she found herself, which was often in open fields. And she carried only what she could fit into the pockets of her tunic: a comb, a folding toothbrush, her mail, a pen, a map,

and, later, copies of her booklet *Steps toward Inner Peace*, which she handed out along her route.

SPEAKING FROM HER HEART

Peace Pilgrim's story is so amazing it's hard to believe that she actually existed. After all, her story seems so incredible: an ordinary woman, hair already turned silver, walking solo across the country (America, no less—land of the automobile), without a penny in her pocket. Yet thousands of newspaper clippings and videos of her lectures vouch for what she was doing.

Peace Pilgrim delivered her speeches like dramatic monologues, raising her eyes to the heavens, waving her arms, clasping and pointing her long, slender fingers to punctuate her message. Clearly, she spoke from her heart, without a trace of judgment or criticism in her words or tone. And she enjoyed herself.

No question could throw Peace Pilgrim off course. No intellectualization could dampen her enthusiasm. She had found inner peace, and she wanted to shout it from the rooftops. "Only as we become peaceful will we find ourselves living in a more peaceful world," she'd say.

To large cities and to small towns, Peace Pilgrim delivered ideas that would eventually become topics in countless books on self-improvement and spiritual development. "Problems are opportunities in disguise" and "Inner peace is where peace begins" were just two of her mantras.

Peace Pilgrim reached out to people not only through the spoken word but also through the written word. During her travels, she corresponded with thousands of people whom she had met and counseled. She also created a newsletter, called *Peace Pilgrim's Progress*, to keep in touch with her friends while on the road.

At the time, what she said seemed radical. Yet she was so compelling, and she so obviously lived by her beliefs, that thousands of people took her into their hearts and even into their homes.

Eventually, Peace Pilgrim found herself inundated with offers of food and shelter. Her problem was no longer waiting to be offered a meal or a place to sleep but finding a way to graciously refuse many of the invitations. Peace Pilgrim had traveled far, literally and figuratively.

REACHING OUT TO EVERYONE

In 1964, when Peace Pilgrim had completed 25,000 miles, she decided to change course. The time had come to stop counting mileage. She had been walking mostly along highways so that she could easily chart her progress. But she wanted to meet more people with whom she could share her message. She decided to visit the towns that she had passed by. There she would find the listeners that she sought.

Along with Peace Pilgrim's change in course came a change in priorities, from walking to speaking. She booked engagements across the country, and she began accepting rides so that she could fit in as many lectures as possible. But she always returned to walking when she had time.

Although Peace Pilgrim believed that people should never look for results from their efforts, she witnessed a change in social and cultural values brought about, at least in part, by her work. In the 1960s, she saw a moral shift away from the belief that war is the answer to conflict. She watched as the fear and apathy of the McCarthy Era gave way to fervent demonstrations for peace. She saw people who had expressed little interest in spiritual growth become hungry for the kind of message that she sought to deliver. The trend toward peace has grown stronger over the years and continues to resonate with all generations.

Peace Pilgrim continued her mission of peace until her death on July 7, 1981. Ironically, she was killed while being driven to a speaking engagement. She left behind no written material other than her newsletters and her booklet *Steps toward Inner Peace.*

When the thousands who followed Peace Pilgrim learned of her death, they joined in spirit to mourn her passing. But we suspect that she would have told them to save their tears. As she said, "The body is just a garment. Death is a glorious transition to a freer life."

In death, Peace Pilgrim was free. But her message lives on.

To learn more about Peace Pilgrim, visit the Web site of the Friends of Peace Pilgrim, www.peacepilgrim.org, or call 203-926-1581. You can request a free copy of *Steps toward Inner Peace* by phone or by e-mail, or you can read it on the Web site.

PART VII

GETTING STARTED WITH DYNAMIC WALKING

INTRODUCTION

Left, right, left, repeat: Walking is such a basic human activity that it seems impossible to improve upon. But there is a system that can help *anyone* get more out of walking, no matter what their speed, fitness level, or health status. It's called *Dynamic Walking*.

Dynamic Walking was developed by Suki Munsell, PhD, a registered movement therapist with extensive experience in the fields of education, psychology, fitness, dance, and somatic studies (a discipline that examines the relationship of the body to thinking, feeling, learning, and healing). She created and developed Dynamic Walking and the Dynamic Body Exercises after 30 years of studying systems of dance and exercise from around the world.

She trains people to walk with grace and efficiency while slowing and perhaps reversing the aging process, preventing injury, and, in many cases, diminishing chronic pain. Using techniques that you'll read about in the next four chapters, she teaches people to modify their habitual movement patterns (their biomechanics) while walking, sitting, standing, and exercising.

Dr. Munsell's approach to fitness has a key element that's absent from most other training programs. She shows her clients how to evaluate their biomechanics to identify the patterns that get in the way of graceful, efficient walking and that may make them vulnerable to injury or delay their healing processes.

Her strategies help restore the body's natural, balanced posture, which enables her clients to walk stronger, faster, and farther. And if her clients do experience any musculoskeletal pain, they're able to heal their bodies and protect themselves against further injury. (Of course, if you have any undiagnosed pain, you should be properly evaluated by a physician before attempting any kind of self-treatment program.)

Dr. Munsell's Dynamic Walking is a unique and effective program that anyone can use. What you are about to learn can turn your daily workout into a source of healing, strength, and vitality.

By moving step-by-step through her techniques, you will learn to walk taller, slimmer, stronger, and longer without discomfort. Read the instructions carefully and apply them daily. You'll marvel at the results!

CHAPTER 32

A NEW WAY OF WALKING

At the Dynamic Health and Fitness Institute in San Anselmo, California, my colleagues and I have developed, refined, and taught a new method of fitness training. Called *Dynamic Walking*, it shows people how to use dynamic forces—such as gravity, momentum, space, time, and intensity—to get more out of their walking workouts and to prevent injuries caused by faulty movement patterns (or biomechanics).

Of course, you already know how to walk. But without realizing it, you may be hampering yourself with poor posture or gait—perhaps because of stress, strain, or injury, or because you're subconsciously imitating the movement patterns of people around you. As you go through the Dynamic Walking program, you'll learn exercises and techniques that can help you develop good biomechanics. You'll be able to walk faster and get a better aerobic workout without creating undue wear and tear on your joints or muscles.

You may have started a walking program to lose weight, to stay healthy, or to improve your fitness. Whatever your reason, Dynamic Walking can help you reach your goal more efficiently and effectively. You'll look and feel great almost instantly as you improve your posture and gait. You'll stay active and have more fun in life, now and for years to come.

THE KEY TO HEALING

One of the greatest advantages of Dynamic Walking is that it helps you protect yourself against the sort of injuries that occur when you perform a certain motion over and over again with poor biomechanics. These are referred to as *repetitive-stress injuries*, and they can occur anywhere in your body. When they're related to exercise, they often show up in the lower back, hips, knees, or feet.

Repetitive-stress injuries are among the many problems that prompt people to come to the Dynamic Health and Fitness Institute for help. Some of our clients have chronic back pain or are recovering from some sort of surgery, and they need to go through a re-education process in order to walk pain free. Other clients are athletes who have suffered injuries that put them back to square one in terms of their training. They use Dynamic Walking as a springboard for resuming their respective sports.

What do all of these people have in common? Invariably, they developed problems in the first place because of faulty movement patterns that created a "weak link" in their bodies, predisposing them to injury. By analyzing each client's posture and stride, I can usually pinpoint a biomechanical cause of the person's pain. That pain is frequently localized in the lower back or on one side of the body or in one joint, such as the knee or hip.

As our clients improve their biome-

chanics, they often experience immediate and long-lasting relief from their discomfort. We have helped many people reduce or eliminate chronic or recurring pain in the back, hips, knees, ankles, feet—even the neck.

Once I teach clients Dynamic Walking, I'll continue to track their progress for several years. Invariably, they report wonderful results. Their postures improve with attention, but without a lot of effort. Their flexibility increases. They're less vulnerable to injury—and if they do hurt themselves, they heal faster. They perform better in other sports, even without practice. Each time they walk dynamically, they reinforce the things I've taught them. Walking dynamically becomes a form of preventive medicine.

My trainers and I also see hundreds of clients who are already pain free and want to stay that way. These people are interested in improving their health and fitness or perhaps losing weight. They want to learn a safe, reliable walking technique to get the best possible workout. Once they complete Dynamic Walking training, they realize that they have gotten much more from it than they originally expected. They understand their bodies much better and are more sensitive to how they look and feel. They have more pride in their appearance, and they derive more pleasure from their walks.

As you progress through the Dynamic Walking program, you can expect similar results. You'll experience dramatic changes in yourself—not only physically but also mentally and emotionally. You'll just feel better inside and out.

THE PSOAS MUSCLES: A KEY COMPONENT OF BALANCED WALKING

You'll notice that many of the exercises and techniques in the Dynamic Walking program target key postural muscles called the psoas. These muscles extend from the bottom of the diaphragm (which separates the chest from the abdomen) to the top of the inside of each thighbone, or femur. The psoas are hip flexors; they're the major muscles doing the work when you bend your chest toward your thighs or pull your knees toward your chest. They also enable you to swing your legs when you walk.

Unfortunately, when you sit a lot, your psoas muscles become tight. They can pull on your spine, increasing its curves and making you shorter. When this happens, you begin to collapse and slump,

which leaves you feeling and looking older. What's more, your breathing becomes shallow, your circulation declines, and many of your muscles and joints don't function properly.

As your psoas muscles tighten, they affect not only your posture but also your gait. They compress your torso so that when you walk, you tend to drop your weight into your hips and land heavily with every step. This causes you to bounce up and down while you're walking, which puts extra stress on your back, hips, and legs. And you take 8,000 to 10,000 steps per day as you go about your daily routine—not even counting your workouts.

With Dynamic Walking, you'll learn to lift out of your hips. This gives your legs room to swing like pendulums, as they are meant to do. (Podiatrists use the term *swing phase* to describe this motion.) The weight of your swinging legs, combined with special stretches called the *Dynamic Body Exercises*, help lengthen your psoas muscles with every step.

POSTURE: THE BENEFITS OF STANDING TALL

Beyond building your psoas muscles, the Dynamic Body Exercises help realign your entire body and strengthen your core. This is key to rebuilding your posture, another objective of the Dynamic Walking program.

Poor posture is a common cause of back pain, which has reached epidemic proportions in the United States. Back pain affects an estimated 80 percent of Americans at some point in their lives. Many of us in the health and fitness industry have devoted years to studying this public health issue. Back pain robs millions of people of their time, money, and enjoyment of life.

In fact, I first developed Dynamic Walking to help heal my own debilitating sciatica. None of the treatment programs that I tried worked for me. So I created my own.

Like many people, I struggled with poor posture. I've had clients tell me that when they were growing up, their mothers (or grandmothers) were constantly trying to get them to stand up straight. Did that happen to you? While your family surely meant well, they likely couldn't tell you *how* to correct your posture effectively. It took me more than 30 years to figure out.

Through Dynamic Walking and the Dynamic Body Exercises, you'll discover a practical approach to achieving good posture. As you practice these techniques, you'll feel better and more relaxed whether you're standing or sitting. That's because you'll learn to allow your skeletal system, not your muscles, to hold you up. Your muscles will be able to let go of unnecessary tension. Your breathing will deepen as your chest has more room to expand.

Improving your posture doesn't have to be a mystery or an effort. But it does take practice. Using the techniques that I've developed makes it a little easier.

GETTING THE MOST FROM DYNAMIC WALKING

When you walk for exercise, your dynamics should precede your aerobics. In other words, before you try to walk fast to get a good workout, you need to learn to walk correctly, with proper posture and stride. If you take poor posture and stride mechanics and add the forces and pressures that speed creates, your body will suffer. With proper biomechanics, you'll be able to walk faster, and you'll feel good while you're doing it. What's more, you'll be able to walk longer at any speed without getting tired or putting yourself at risk for injury.

In Chapter 33, I'll guide you through a 6-week program in which you'll examine your habitual movement patterns and learn techniques for correcting your posture and stride. Even if you have been fitness walking for years, you need to analyze your biomechanics in this way. Once you do, you're ready to learn to walk dynamically. Anyone with a chronic condition, such as diabetes, should talk with their doctors before beginning this—or any—exercise program.

In Chapter 34, I'll teach you the Dynamic Body Exercises, which you'll begin practicing during the 6-week program. The Dynamic Body Exercises go hand in hand with Dynamic Walking. The exercises stretch and rebalance your musculoskeletal system. Then Dynamic Walking "sets" your new posture and stride. If you try to master the walking technique without doing the exercises, you won't get the results you want.

Unfortunately, in the rush to get through their workouts, few people stretch regularly, correctly, or completely. Done carefully and consistently, stretching feels great and helps you maintain your flexibility as you grow older or exercise harder. The Dynamic Body Exercises can help you discover the joys of stretching. They can be done before, after, and even during a walking workout.

In Chapter 35, you'll learn a Dynamic Walking routine to use every time you walk. It's designed with respect for your body's natural timing in warming up, cooling down, and stretching. Built into the routine are awareness exercises to help you monitor your progress and keep your workouts safe.

I recommend completing the 6-week program before starting the Dynamic Walking routine. That way, you can concentrate on developing correct posture and stride, then apply those skills to walking dynamically.

As we move on with your Dynamic Walking training, please remember to ease yourself into this or any fitness program, especially if you have been inactive. On the first day, do only half as much as you think you can. Progress gradually from there.

You may experience some soreness from time to time; this is to be expected as you retrain your body to move in different, more efficient ways. If any pain persists or gets worse, by all means see your doctor. Once your doctor rules out any underlying medical problem, you can continue with the Dynamic Walking program.

CHAPTER 33

6 WEEKS TO DYNAMIC WALKING

Welcome to the start of a 6-week program in which you'll learn and practice the three core principles of the Dynamic Walking program. Through the exercises and techniques in this chapter, you'll do the following:

- **Lift**—lengthen your spine and pull up from your hips and your lower back.
- **Stack**—correct your postural alignment, repositioning the building blocks of your body.
- **Build pelvic power**—energize your walk from your pelvis by connecting strongly to the ground through your legs.

Over the next 6 weeks, you'll be working from the top of your body down toward your feet, then back up. The order is critical to your progress.

In weeks 1 and 2, you'll learn how to *lift* your upper-body weight out of your midsection and your hips. This lift, or decompression, creates more space for your legs to swing like pendulums. The swinging motion, in turn, evenly lengthens and strengthens your psoas muscles. These muscles run down each side of your body, from the base of your diaphragm to the tops of your thighs.

As explained in Chapter 32, the psoas muscles are often tight from too much sitting. This can shorten your posture, limit your breathing, and painfully strangle your sciatic nerve.

But as the psoas muscles become longer and stronger, they're able to maintain your pelvis in a neutral position, which is critical in providing postural support for your torso and upper body.

The combination of decompressing and psoas-lengthening makes it easier to *stack*, or realign, the building blocks of your body—that is, your head, chest, pelvis, hips, and legs. In weeks 3 and 4, you'll learn to assess your posture and make any necessary adjustments.

Relieving your hips of upper-body pressure also allows your legs to change their structural alignment, the focus of week 5. Your legs are the foundation of efficient and effortless posture. They must support everything above them, *and* they must move your body around. With Dynamic Walking, your legs will do a better job of providing both stability and action for your body.

In week 6, you'll *build pelvic power* by connecting from your torso through your legs into the Earth. Your ground traction will improve, and your legs will grow stronger. You'll also decrease upper-body tension and effort as you trust your legs to do their work. In Chapter 35, you'll be adding the power of your arm swing.

THE DYNAMICS OF CHANGE

If you need more than 6 weeks to develop a solid foundation for Dynamic Walking, please be patient with yourself. After all, your current walk has evolved over the course of your lifetime. Changing such a fundamental pattern can seem overwhelming. It's quite normal to feel confused, awkward, and uncoordinated.

Respect the fact that you're making changes in the deepest level of your being, your neurological programming. Be compassionate and persistent, as if training a puppy, and give yourself the time that you need. Even 8 to 12 weeks is reasonable, and you'll be delighted with the results.

Remember, you are deeply identified with your walk and your posture. It's your choice to change them, and you can do so only when you are truly ready. I had one client tell me that correcting his posture made him feel disconnected from his father and grandfather, who also stood with rounded shoulders. Many women say that they first started slumping when their breasts began developing, because they were embarrassed. The human ego has its reasons for wanting to maintain the status quo.

On the other hand, pain is a great motivator for making postural changes. Staying young and vital is another. By progressing slowly and steadily, you allow yourself time to adjust to feeling taller, sexier, or more alive.

Perhaps the most powerful incentive for making the changes that I'm recommending is the increased pleasure derived from moving your body in a smooth, fluid manner, and not just while walking. To help you focus your efforts, I've included with each week's exercises a list of goals as well as a set of what I call kinesthetic images. Remember, to really transform your body, you must develop a new kinesthetic awareness—that is, a new sense of how your body moves.

BUILDING BETTER BIOMECHANICS

When you're ready to begin the program, think of it as performing an experiment for 6 weeks (or however long you need). Your body may feel uncomfortable on occasion as things shift around. Some of my clients have opted to stop other forms of exercise, especially weight training, during this time. Why work against yourself by strengthening muscles in the wrong position? Give your body time to realign itself before adding more stress.

As soon as you start week I of the program, you may also begin stretching dynamically, as described in Chapter 34. If your exercise routine already includes stretching, you need to know that the way you're stretching is part of your habitual movement pattern. It is keeping you in the posture you have now. Think about that. You'll get faster results if you stop your other stretches for a while and do the Dynamic Body Exercises (DBX) correctly and completely. You'll learn biomechanical principles that you can then apply to everything you do, from gardening to driving a car. (*Biomechanics* refers to your body movement patterns.)

During each week of the 6-week program, I'll ask you to focus on specific Dynamic Body Exercises, practicing them in conjunction with other exercises. By targeting specific aspects of posture and stride, they'll systematically transform your body.

Transforming your body can be an exciting project, like redesigning a room in your home. Keep in mind that your posture affects not only how you carry your weight but also how you look, feel, age, and heal. Watch for these positive changes as you progress through the program.

Knowledge is power. More power to you.

WEEK 1: LIFTING YOUR UPPER BODY

If you notice these signs: C- or S-shaped posture—slumping, collapsed chest, shoulders rolled forward, shallow breathing, bulging belly, swayback; pain in the lower back, hips, buttocks, knees, or heels; feeling like life is an uphill battle

You'll practice these exercises: Side Stroke; Short Shirt Pull; DBX Focus

You'll experience these benefits: Feeling lighter and taller; breathing more fully; experiencing more comfort and less pain; feeling that you've lost weight; being happier

You'll achieve this training goal: Lifting your upper-body weight out of your midsection and lower back

Perhaps you've heard the word *psychosomatic*. It means that your feelings can profoundly affect your body. Indeed, research has shown that negative feelings can produce illness.

The opposite is also true. Alexander Lowen, an early mind–body researcher, discovered that the set (posture) of the soma (body) affects the psyche. He coined the term *somatopsychic*.

You can test Lowen's theory for yourself by doing the following exercise. Begin to slump as you sit reading this book. Continue slumping. Imagine how you'll look in 5 years, in 10 years. How has your breathing changed? How do you feel? What would your life be like if this was your posture? What activities would you have to give up? What would happen to you if you couldn't straighten up? Scary thought, isn't it?

Your body position quite literally affects your outlook on life. Renowned psychiatrist Sigmund Freud once said, "Anatomy is destiny." Perhaps both he and Lowen were warning us that, all too easily, our biology can become our biography.

I've heard it said that while we can't always determine our future, we can determine our habits. Our habits determine our future.

If you experience any of the warning signals listed above, or if you want to avoid them, then practice the following exercises and techniques to decompress your spine. You'll get more lift out of life.

Exercises for Week 1

Repeat these frequently each day this week to build new muscle memory.

Side Stroke. While standing, place your

right hand at your left side. Beneath your hand, feel the distance between your rib cage and your hip. Then inhale as you stretch your left arm upward, lifting out of your waist. Feel how you can increase the distance beneath your hand.

Now as you exhale, lower your left shoulder and arm, but maintain that increased space beneath your hand. You're training the muscles around your rib cage to keep you lifted. This will give you more breathing space and reduce the pressure on your lower back. Repeat three times on each side.

Short Shirt Pull. Cross your arms at the wrists and position them at about waist height. Raise your arms overhead, as if pulling off a shirt. Inhale fully, stretching your arms overhead. Lengthen your torso as you reach toward the sky. Resist the urge to arch your back. Keep your head level, with your gaze fixed on the horizon. Exhale and return your arms to your sides while continuing to grow taller through your spine.

Repeat the exercise. Make sure that as you lower your arms, you drop your shoulders like a shirt resting on a hanger. Repeat several more times, imagining that you're pulling off your old body to reveal a lighter, brighter you.

The next time you go walking, do three to six Short Shirt Pulls every few minutes. Notice how the movement alters your walk. Resume your "old" walk and feel the difference.

Practice the exercise frequently during your walking workouts this week, so you retain the lifted posture. Also do a Short Shirt Pull whenever you catch yourself slumping. Don't criticize yourself for slouching; instead, congratulate yourself for being aware of your posture and correcting it.

DBX Focus. Learn how to do the Long Shirt Pull exercise described on page 234.

Kinesthetic Images for Week 1

Practice these frequently each day this week to experience your body in new ways.

Crowning Glory. Lift your head high into an imaginary crown. Balance your head gently at the top of your spine. Make sure that your ears are positioned over your shoulders. Relax your jaw, and relax your face.

Shoulder Shirt. Let your shoulders relax and drop. Imagine them hanging like a shirt on a hanger.

Growing Upward. Whenever you see a

tree rising straight and tall into the sky or a flower poised at the end of a slender upright stalk or a person moving with elegant lifted posture, bring that experience into your own body. Imagine that you're riding an upward energy that lifts your body and spirit skyward.

Home Base. Do a Short Shirt Pull. As your arms come down, relax your shoulders completely. Add several Shoulder Rolls (page 237)—up, back, down, and around—to settle your shoulders like a yoke resting easily on your rib cage. Let the weight of your arms help keep your shoulders relaxed.

Feel the core of your body supporting you. Close your eyes and allow your body to lead you through some spontaneous stretches. This helps you find home base, a comfortable position where your muscles relax and your skeleton supports you.

Goals for Week 1

1. Walk for 10 to 30 minutes, 3 to 5 times this week, while maintaining an elongated spine.
2. Do 10 to 20 Short Shirt Pulls during each of your walking workouts. Also practice the Short Shirt Pulls

frequently during the day to help build and maintain a lifted posture. You're strengthening the levatores costarum muscles, which raise your ribs, to maintain lift.

3. Become aware of when you are lifted and when you are slumping forward.
4. Acknowledge yourself each time you catch yourself in an old habit and you make a positive change.
5. Keep your shoulders relaxed and down while standing taller through your spine.
6. Notice differences in how you carry your weight and how you look and feel.

WEEK 2: LIFTING OUT OF YOUR HIPS

If you notice these signs: Tightness or pain in the lower back or hips; heaviness in the abdomen; shallow breathing; knee or foot pain; slow pace when walking; less get-up-and-go

You'll practice these exercises: Pendulum Arms; Pendulum Legs—Scuff/No Scuff; Nose over Toes to Go; DBX Focus

You'll experience these benefits: Feeling lighter on your feet; walking faster and easier; developing greater flexibility; breathing easier; improving digestion and elimination; feeling more vital and alive

You'll achieve this training goal: Lifting your upper-body weight out of your hips

In week 1, you began learning to send your energy up your spine while leaving your shoulders down and relaxed. Your goals included building important new habits: training the levatores costarum (the muscles that raise your ribs) to maintain lift and training yourself to assume a taller posture whenever you find yourself slumping.

In week 2, you'll be lifting your body up out of your hips. This will create enough space to move your legs like pendulums. Why is this important? Well, have you ever pushed a child on a swing? A swing is a pendulum. After those first few pushes, it moves by itself, with little additional effort to keep it going. The swing moves efficiently because it uses momentum, which is a dynamic force.

You can learn to use momentum to fuel your walk and save energy. You have four pendulums—two arms and two legs—attached to your body. The tricky part is letting go of the tension you may habitually hold in your shoulders and your hips so that your limbs can swing freely. Ninety-five percent of the people whom I watch walk are not swinging their legs. Instead, they're stepping forward, reaching forward, or falling onto their feet and legs.

Watch for yourself how people walk. Steppers, reachers, and fallers bounce up and down; they're using their leg muscles as springs. The people who swing their legs are gliding. Their walk is smooth at any speed, slow or fast. My husband, Russ, who developed our Dynamic Speed program, has been clocked at an 8$\frac{1}{2}$-minute-per-mile pace. And his walk is smooth, never bobbing.

Unless you are among the 5 percent of people who naturally swing their legs like pendulums, Dynamic Walking will be dramatically different for you. The glide feels great, it looks great, it's dynamic. Best of all, it's less jarring to your joints. Since you're averaging 8,000 steps a day, plus 2,000 more for every mile of fitness walking you do, that jarring adds up fast.

Swinging your arms and legs uses

dynamic forces wisely. It is economical. You won't be wasting your energy. As a result, you may notice that you can walk farther.

Walking dynamically is a metaphor for learning to use natural resources with more awareness and respect. You'll also be learning to use your muscles differently, so initially you may notice soreness in new places.

Exercises for Week 2

Repeat these as needed each day this week to build new muscle memory. Be sure to practice the first three exercises every time you go fitness walking, until you feel yourself gliding easily. If it seems difficult or confusing, don't get discouraged, and don't try too hard. Relaxing into the glide is key.

Pendulum Arms. Stand tall. Bend forward from your hips as if to place both hands on a table. Let your arms hang limp. Reach over with your right hand and push your left arm only once. Let your arm swing until it stops. Do it again. Continue releasing any tension in your left shoulder until your arm is totally relaxed and swinging easily. Describe to yourself how your shoulder feels. Compare as you repeat the exercise with your right arm.

Each time you go fitness walking, let your arms swing relaxed at your sides for at least 10 minutes. Don't pump them or use them to power your walk—not yet, anyway.

Pendulum Legs—Scuff/No Scuff. Begin with a Short Shirt Pull. Then, while you're standing tall, place your right hand on a support (such as a wall or the back of a sturdy, stable chair) and balance on your right leg. Breathe as you rhythmically swing your left leg back and forth several times from the hip joint. Keep both knees relaxed.

Scuff your left foot on the ground several times as you swing. Then swing without scuffing. Repeat the Scuff/No Scuff twice more. Notice that lifting out of your right hip socket allows your left leg to swing freely and clear the ground. When you scuff the ground, you're settling into your right hip socket. Describe to yourself how your right hip feels. Compare as you repeat the exercise while standing on your left leg.

To transfer this exercise to walking, position yourself with your left side toward a long wall or railing. Practice swinging your right leg (from the hip, not the knee) like a relaxed pendulum. To ensure that you are doing the exercise correctly, reach down with your right hand to pump your leg a few times. If your hip is relaxed, your leg should respond as if you are pushing a swing. Swing your right foot gently into place just ahead of your left foot. This will be shorter than your normal stride length. Step onto your right foot, rolling heel to toe.

Switch sides and repeat the exercise with your left leg. Be careful not to pound your heel. Repeat several more times, alternating legs as you go.

Nose over Toes to Go. Stand with your feet parallel and about one shoe-width apart. Do a Short Shirt Pull. To initiate your first step, lean forward from your ankles—not your hips—until your nose is over your toes. This lean positions your legs under and slightly to the rear of your body. Push off from behind with your right leg, allowing it to swing forward, relaxed from the hip, into the Heel-Toe Roll (page 234). Don't think about stepping forward. Concentrate only on the push-off from the ball and toes of the foot that is to the rear of your body.

After your first step, you don't need to continue leaning forward. Do Short Shirt Pulls whenever you're walking, to stand tall and stay lifted out of your hips.

If you sink back into your pelvis, you will naturally return to a bouncy stride. If you practice walking dynamically during the day, you'll notice faster results.

DBX Focus. You'll know you've succeeded in releasing shoulder tension when your arms drop and flop at your sides during the Spinal Rotation (page 239). Also practice letting your arms dangle while you're doing Shoulder Rolls (page 237) and the Hamstring Stretch (page 241).

Kinesthetic Images for Week 2

Practice these often each day this week to experience your body in new ways.

Limp Limbs. Have you seen someone holding a sleeping child? The child's body, arms, and legs are limp. While you're in bed, practice letting your arms and legs go limp. You may need to squeeze your muscles tight a few times, then relax them with a strong exhale. Proceed up your body, from the muscles in your feet to those in your head. (This exercise, called *progressive muscle relaxation*, is excellent for releasing tension.) Anchor this new feeling in your body. Think of it as hitting the R key (for "relax") on your "bio-computer." Transfer this new kinesthetic image into your everyday life.

Pendulum Arms and Legs. Have you ever seen a child spin around in a circle, her arms following her body? When you're walking, let your arms swing as a result of your movement. Let your legs swing forward passively as a result of your push-off.

Goals for Week 2

1. Lift out of your hips.
2. Swing your legs forward like pendulums as you walk.
3. Relax your hips and the muscles of your pelvic floor.
4. Allow your arms to swing relaxed from your shoulders while you're walking.
5. Increase your daily awareness of tension in your shoulders and your hips. Inhale, exhale, and let tension dissolve.

WEEK 3: ASSESSING YOUR POSTURE FROM THE MIDLINE

If you notice these signs: Backaches; hip, spine, or leg pain

You'll practice these exercises: Dynamic Posture Analysis—Midline; DBX Focus; Dynamic Stride Analysis—Midline; Dynamic Walking Training

You'll experience these benefits: Having less pain; feeling more relaxed and less tense; experiencing less muscle strain; developing better balance; getting a better workout; enjoying more confidence; looking better

You'll achieve this training goal: Improving postural alignment from the front or midline

When infants first begin to sit upright on their own, they hold their spines ramrod straight. Their legs are also straight, extended wide to help create a stable, triangular base. They sit on the floor this way when stacking blocks or dropping colorful rings onto an upright post. Perhaps this is how they learn to stack the building blocks of their bodies before attempting to walk.

During week 2, your task was to incorporate a new awareness—to separate your core from your arms and legs, which can then hang relaxed when you're standing still or swing when you're in motion. To accomplish this, I asked you to continue lifting your torso upward, all the way out of your hips.

This allows your legs to swing like pendulums when you walk.

What's more, the upward energy decompresses and elongates your spine, which allows the building blocks of your body to shift more easily into a biomechanically efficient posture. So your posture better supports you while you're at rest and as you move through your daily activities.

This week, you'll analyze your daily biomechanics and connect this awareness to your walking biomechanics. As an example, one woman came to me with pain in her right hip that was so severe she couldn't even put on her panty hose. She had sought help from several doctors, but they couldn't tell her what was wrong. After studying her posture in photographs, she realized that she was rotated to her right and sinking (compressed) into her right hip. All day long, she was managing a team of people whose desks were to her right and behind her. With her new awareness, plus walking and stretching dynamically, she relieved her pain.

Have you ever wanted x-ray vision, like Superman? Well, I can't grant you that, but I can teach you to "see" bodies with a greater awareness of the structure that lies beneath.

For example, if your fanny pack, waist belt, or socks are twisting around when you walk, you are probably pushing off harder on one foot. If your shoes wear unevenly, you're likely dealing with unbalanced biomechanics.

Looking at a herd of zebras, you'd have a hard time telling the animals apart as individuals. Their shape and movements make them look almost identical. They must move with respect to dynamic forces to avoid becoming some lion's dinner. It is the law of survival of the fittest. Poor biomechanics might cost zebras their lives. For us humans, it may only reduce the length and quality of life.

The next exercise is the toughest so far. It requires you to look at yourself in a full-length mirror. If you don't already have such a mirror, consider buying one. They're inexpensive and easy to store. You'll need one to track your progress.

I want you to see beyond your immediate reaction to how you look—too heavy, too slumped, too something. Drop all that. Pretend that you have x-ray vision. Look deeper into your musculoskeletal structure.

Exercises for Week 3

Repeat these as needed each day this week to develop new muscle memory.

Dynamic Posture Analysis—Midline. Hang a weighted string down the center of a full-length mirror. Then position yourself in front of the mirror so that you can view your body from head to toe. Find your natural standing posture.

Using the string for reference, observe your body. Does the center line fall straight from your nose to your belly button to between your feet? Do you lean to one side? Do you put more weight on one leg? Is an arm longer, a hip higher, a shoulder lower? Is the space between your arms and your body the same on both sides? Does your clothing wrinkle unevenly or hang differently from one side of your body to the other?

Stand for about a minute, until you feel your body getting tired. Close your eyes and notice in which direction you would most easily shift, twist, or collapse to relieve tightness or tension. Open your eyes and watch closely as you move back and forth between postures. Notice whether different postures make you feel differently about yourself.

Relieve any tension that may have built up from standing by proceeding to the next exercise.

DBX Focus. Do three Long Shirt Pulls (page 234). Begin each one with a Heel-Toe Roll (page 234) to distribute your weight more evenly between your legs. As you roll up, pay attention to how you stack your pelvis over your legs, align your rib cage over your pelvis, settle your shoulder yoke on your rib cage, and perch your head atop your spinal column.

Over the next few weeks, pay attention to the changes you see in the mirror. Close your eyes and feel what has changed. Transfer this new awareness into your everyday life.

Dynamic Stride Analysis—Midline. Whenever you go walking, pay attention to the following (you may want to tape-record these points, so you don't have to memorize them).

- Feet and legs: Look down to observe whether your feet are tracking parallel or pointing in or out. Can you see or feel that you are collapsing to the inside or outside of your feet? Are you on one leg for a longer period than the other? Does one push off harder or step out farther? If you have any pain, analyze which part of your movement hurts.

- Hips: Walk with your hands on your hips, thumbs pointing forward. Notice whether both hips are moving the same or at all. Drop your hands to your sides.
- Arms: Place one hand on your chest for 15 paces. Observe the power of the arm that is swinging. Then change hands for 15 paces. Does one arm seem stronger or more dominant than the other? Switch hands again, this time concentrating on your arm position. Does one arm swing more easily to the front or back? Or do your arms swing equally in both directions? Continue switching until you have a good comparison of the power and tracking of both arms.
- Back: Bring both hands toward your chest as if you are carrying a package. How does this change your walk? Do you experience pain in your lower back? Drop your arms.
- Head: Notice where you tend to look when you walk. Do you feel any strain in your neck, shoulders, or upper back?

When you are finished, choose three words to describe your most vivid impression of your walk.

Dynamic Walking Training. Whenever you go walking, use your stride analysis to make observations about your body. If one arm swings forward more easily and the other swings back more easily, perhaps your body is rotated. If you feel more weight on one leg, perhaps you're subconsciously favoring that leg or leaning to that side. Your goal is to begin using both sides of your body more evenly when you walk, stand, and exercise.

As you're walking, make the following changes:

- Feet and legs: Walk with your feet pointing straight ahead. Push off equally from the balls and toes of both feet. If one or both of your feet angle out to the sides, practice keeping them parallel for only 1 to 2 minutes at a time, 3 to 5 times during your walk. Gradually increase the duration and frequency over the next 3 to 9 months, until you're able to hold your feet in a parallel position without discomfort.
- Hips: Once you're more lifted, the weight of your swinging legs will naturally swivel your hips. Holding back your hips or forcing the swivel causes strain. Just continue to do Short Shirt Pulls while you walk and let nature take its course.
- Arms: Let your arms swing forward and back equally, like pendulums. (In

Chapter 35, you'll learn the bent-arm technique.)

- Head: Keep your head level, gently perched atop your spine. Let your eyes scan the path ahead of you far to near for safety. As you do the Short Shirt Pulls (10 to 20 per hour), maintain a lift into your crown.
- Breathing: Let your breathing relax. As you continue to elongate your spine, your breaths will deepen.

Kinesthetic Image for Week 3

Practice this frequently each day this week to experience your body in new ways.

Balloon Breathing. As you breathe, notice which area of your body moves. Then empty your lungs by exhaling forcefully. Often we don't let go of "old" air, so we don't have room for fresh air. As you inhale, imagine your torso filling fully all around, like a balloon. Exhale fully and pause. You'll notice that your body inhales on its own when it needs air. Repeat several times.

Goals for Week 3

1. Be more aware of how you use your body in everyday activities.

2. Stack the building blocks of your body in better alignment.
3. Use both sides of your body more symmetrically when you walk, stand, and exercise.
4. Use your full-length mirror to observe your posture.

WEEK 4: ASSESSING YOUR POSTURE FROM THE SIDE

If you notice these signs: Headaches; eyestrain; shoulder tension; shallow breathing; backaches; hip, spine, or leg pain; poor circulation; depression

You'll practice these exercises: Dynamic Posture Analysis—Plumb Line; Belly Button to Backbone with Heel Press; Psoas Heel Slide; Rib Cage Slide; DBX Focus

You'll experience these benefits: Improving posture; enjoying greater comfort; having less pain; breathing deeper; feeling more relaxed and less tense; experiencing less muscle strain; improving balance; working out more effectively; striding with confidence; looking better

You'll achieve this training goal: Improving postural alignment from the side or plumb line

Several years ago, our local newspaper ran an article on the design of shirts to fit the body of the average older woman. Typically, her shoulders have rolled forward, and her rib cage sits on her hips. This posture is unfortunate and unnecessary, most likely brought on by a combination of poor biomechanics and the brittle-bone disease osteoporosis.

Proper nutrition, weight training, and hormonal balance can prevent osteoporosis. Likewise, good biomechanics can prevent collapse. Whether you're a woman or a man, standing tall communicates to the world your self-respect at any age.

The upright posture is highly valued in cultures worldwide. It's captured in the cave paintings of warriors, the tomb paintings of Egyptian pharaohs, the statues of Greek gods, the erect spine of Buddha, the regal bearings of kings and queens. In the animated film *Mulan*, which is about a young Chinese woman impersonating a man in battle, she prays to bring honor to her family so that her father "can stand tall." In the English language, we refer to people as "upstanding citizens."

Last week, you began to take a deeper look at yourself, to assess how you're growing your body. (As the twig is bent, the saying goes, so the tree will grow.) This week, you'll analyze your posture from the side. You'll need to have a friend take photos of you. It's impossible to use a mirror effectively.

You'll continue to concentrate on stacking the building blocks of your body more efficiently. To do this, you'll learn an exercise to lengthen and strengthen the psoas muscles, which are located deep in your abdomen and connect your spine to your legs.

As you analyze your posture, maintaining a positive attitude can make all the difference. None of us is perfect. We all see things in ourselves that we could correct. Your goal is to correct poor biomechanics. That's different from deciding that you or some part of your body is "bad" or "wrong." Stop saying "my bad leg" or "my bad knee." That only adds insult to injury. It's counterproductive.

Instead, build a more positive, more nurturing vocabulary. Use words like "previously injured" or "recovering." One leg or arm may be "more dominant" or "less dominant" than the other. Parts of your body may be "overburdened" or "underutilized." You may be "carrying more weight" than you want to. Your movement patterns may be "untrained" or "inefficient."

Choose your words carefully and with compassion. They have the power to launch a war or nurture love, to kill or create. Ultimately, they affect your thoughts, your feelings about yourself, and your posture.

Respect your body for the extraordinary gift that it is, and thank it for bringing you this far.

Exercises for Week 4

Repeat these as instructed to build new muscle memory.

Dynamic Posture Analysis—Plumb Line. Stand as you would at the end of the day, perhaps even closing your eyes to feel the posture you want to have captured on film. Then have a friend take a photo of you from each side. Looking at the pictures, place a dot on your ear, shoulder, hip, knee, and ankle. Connect the dots to see if they're in a straight line, perpendicular to the floor, or if they form a C or an S curve.

Now look carefully at your posture. Are your ears over your shoulders, or is your head forward? Are your shoulders over your hips? Is your upper body slightly behind your lower body, the way a model might walk with her hips pushed forward? Is your back swayed? Is your waistband parallel to the ground or slanted?

Draw a box around your pelvis, using your waistband as the top of the box. Does your pelvic bowl spill forward, creating a belly bulge? Are your knees locked?

Roll down into a Long Shirt Pull (page 234). As you roll up, experiment with restacking the building blocks of your body into better alignment. Repeat twice more. This teaches you how to make your skeletal system bear more of your body weight and how to let your muscles relax. Repeat the Long Shirt Pull frequently throughout the day to maintain lift and spinal flexibility.

Once you've analyzed your photos, label and date them, then store them away for future reference. Some of my clients have new photos taken every 3 to 6 months so that they can see their progress.

If you notice in your photos that you have a C- or an S-shaped posture, practice the following three exercises twice each day this week to build new muscle memory.

Belly Button to Backbone with Heel Press. This floor exercise helps release and lengthen core postural muscles.

Lie on your back on the floor, with your knees bent. Use a towel or pillow to support your neck and head, if necessary. Take a few moments to breathe and let your body melt into the floor. Bring your fingertips to your waist to help you notice the space between your lower back and the floor. To close this space, exhale and press your belly button toward your backbone. Press your heels into the floor to hold this position. Remember the connection between feeling your lower back against the floor and pressing your heels against the floor. Breathe in fully and let the space between your lower back and the floor open up again.

Repeat this exercise several more times, pressing your belly button to your backbone and your heels into the floor on each exhale and releasing on each inhale. Enjoy the rocking motion of your pelvis. Notice which muscles in your torso seem to be working. Don't tighten your abdominal muscles; keep your belly relaxed.

Identify and begin using deeper muscles, especially your psoas. These are your core postural muscles. Stay on the floor and move on to the next exercise.

Psoas Heel Slide. In this exercise, your eventual goal is to straighten both legs while keeping your belly button pressed toward your backbone and your heels pressed into the floor. If you are sway-backed, this will be very difficult at first. Your lower back and psoas muscles may already have shortened. That's what happened to me.

You're still lying on the floor, with your knees bent. On the exhale, slide your left heel *along the floor*, away from your left buttock. Keep your right knee bent, with your right foot comfortably close to your right buttock. Can you continue pressing your lower back against the floor while your left leg is straight?

Bend your left knee, bringing your foot toward your left buttock. Then repeat the exercise, this time extending your right leg by sliding your right heel forward. What happens to your lower back?

Continue alternating legs, sliding one heel and then the other away from your buttocks. Roll your head from side to side, as needed, to keep your neck, shoulders, and upper back relaxed. Breathe deeply; focus on slowly stretching and lengthening the muscles along your back and deep inside your torso.

Always do this exercise with the Belly Button to Backbone with Heel Press. Together, they should take you 3 to 5 minutes. If you have a severe C or S curve to your posture, be sure to do both exercises at least twice a day. Always follow them with the Rib Cage Slide.

Rib Cage Slide. When you carry something, be it a package or a baby, you're likely to push your rib cage too far back behind your lower body. If this posture becomes a habit, it can compress nerves over time, resulting in lower-back and sciatic pain.

If you noticed in your photos that your upper back may be behind your hips, be sure to concentrate on this exercise. It will teach you to move your rib cage into proper position, building a more efficient postural pattern.

The Rib Cage Slide has three parts. First, while standing in front of a full-length mirror, put your hands on either side of your body and extend your fingers so that you're reaching from your lower ribs to your hips. Hold this position while you look in the mirror. Notice where you usually carry your rib cage in relationship to your pelvis.

Next, lie on the floor with your knees bent and your lower back pressed into the floor, as in the Belly Button to Backbone exercise. Again, place your hands at your sides, extending your fingers from your lower ribs to your hips. Notice any difference? The floor is forcing your rib cage more to the front of your pelvis, compared with when you're standing.

Return to a standing position, again noticing where you carry your rib cage. Do a Long Shirt Pull (page 234) to elongate your body. Then do a Heel-Toe Roll (page 234), pausing when you're back on your heels. Bring your belly button toward your backbone, as though you were pressing into the floor. Feel how this simultaneously slides your rib cage forward. (If you want, extend your fingers at your sides to check this new position.) You need only a slight movement; don't try to lift up your rib cage in front, which would cause you to overarch your back. Continue relaxed breathing as you hold this position for 15 seconds.

Repeat the Heel-Toe Roll for 15 seconds, swinging your arms while you do. Then once again pause with your weight back on your heels. Repeat the Belly Button to Backbone exercise and the Rib Cage Slide. Lengthen your lower back, as though you have a heavy tail that's dropping toward the floor. Do the entire sequence a third time. To release any tension that may have built up in your back, do a Hip Stretch (page 240).

Practice the Rib Cage Slide whenever you notice that your rib cage has dropped back and down. Eventually, as your musculoskeletal system adjusts, this new posture will feel more natural.

DBX Focus. If your posture analysis shows you that your upper body is positioned behind your lower body, then from here on, follow every Long and Short Shirt Pull you do with a Belly Button to Backbone exercise and a Rib Cage Slide. You also need to practice lifting your chin slightly.

Use this new postural alignment whenever you are stretching or walking. If your speed increases slightly while you're walking, then you'll know that you were probably pushing your hips forward before.

Kinesthetic Images for Week 4

Practice these frequently each day this week to experience your body in new ways.

Strong Center Core. If you noticed in your photo that you have a C- or an S-shaped posture, then practicing the Belly Button to Backbone exercise and the Rib Cage Slide will bring your body's building blocks into better alignment. Find a positive image to which you can anchor this new kinesthetic awareness, perhaps a classic Greek column or a redwood tree or even a strong wire coil.

Tail Drop. Elongate your spine from your neck to your lower back. Imagine that you have a heavy tail dropping down toward the ground. If you tend to overarch your back, try wearing a fanny pack with a little extra weight when you walk. When I do this, it reminds me to keep my tail down.

Goals for Week 4

1. After a great workout, close your eyes and notice how good you feel. Give this feeling a name and recall it frequently. This helps anchor in your mind a positive new image of your body.
2. Become more aware of your body language.
3. Notice how your posture affects your mood.
4. Choose the appropriate postures throughout your day to achieve your goals, just as you would choose the

appropriate wardrobe to be most effective and comfortable.

WEEK 5: EVALUATING YOUR LEGS

If you notice these signs: Bunions; heel spurs; ankle, knee, or hip pain; iliotibial pain (along the outer thigh); lower-back pain; poor posture

You'll practice these exercises: Shoe Check; Shoe Shopping; Dynamic Posture Analysis—Base (Feet to Hips); Ladder Base into Heel-Toe Roll (or Modified Heel-Toe Roll); DBX Focus

You'll experience these benefits: Increasing comfort; decreasing pain and muscle strain; improving balance; striding with greater ease and strength

You'll achieve this training goal: Improving posture, beginning in your feet

The legs connect the torso with the Earth. Without them, we wouldn't have traction on the ground, and we couldn't walk. Often, however, we locate our awareness in our heads and pay little attention to our lower extremities.

Still, we demand a lot from our legs. They hold us up, and over the course of an average lifetime, they carry us some 115,000 miles—more than four times around the circumference of the globe. Fitness walkers, hikers, and runners rack up even more mileage.

We assume that our legs are ready to go anywhere, anytime. We rarely stretch them properly before moving them. Some of us carry extra loads in our work and extra pounds on our bodies. Or we wear poor-fitting shoes. In fact, we probably think more about our cars than about our legs. We don't service our legs unless they complain, and it surprises us when they do.

Have you ever watched a dance performance—perhaps a ballroom competition or a ballet—and marveled at the strength and precision of the dancers' legs? It took years of dance training before my legs were no longer mere workhorses.

In previous weeks, you learned to lighten the load on your legs and to rebalance the upper-body weight that they must carry. This helps them support you and transport you more efficiently.

Posture begins in your feet. So does powerful walking. When you walk, the most natural biomechanical movement is to roll from heel to toe. Your heel lands slightly to the outside, and you push off between your big toe and second toe. So you're rolling not down the exact centerline of each foot but in a gentle curve from the outside of the heel toward the inside of the ball.

This week, you'll analyze your lower quadrant—your hips and legs, your knees and feet—to discover how to improve your walking biomechanics. This will add miles to your life and joy to your miles.

Exercises for Week 5

Repeat these as instructed.

Shoe Check. Take out your oldest pair of walking shoes and look at the soles. Bare patches on the soles show where you exert pressure. Is the tread worn differently from one shoe to the other? Is it worn unevenly from left to right on each shoe? This information tells a story about how you use your body.

Next, place your shoes on a table and look at them from the front. Is one toebox creased or crumpled differently than the other? Bend down so that you can view your shoes at eye level from the back. Are they different heights? If one shoe appears flatter than the other, it means you're carrying more body weight on that leg.

Connect this information with what you learned from your stride analysis and posture analysis in weeks 3 and 4. Each time you buy new walking shoes, take a moment to check your old shoes. It's another way to monitor your biomechanics to be sure that you're using proper form.

If you wear orthotics (specially designed shoe inserts), you might want to remove them for short periods—say, 10 to 20 minutes—during your workouts. This gives your musculoskeletal system a chance to realign itself. If you don't have any pain, you can gradually reduce the amount of time you're wearing orthotics, either while walking or while going about your daily activities. This systematic approach to weaning off orthotics was suggested to me by my colleague Harry Hlavac, DPM, a biomechanicist and author of *The Foot Book*.

Shoe Shopping. Unless your shoes are less than 2 months old and still fresh, buy new ones this week. The old pair is worn in a postural pattern that will keep you from making the changes you desire. Buying new ones will help you put your best foot forward. Find a shoe salesperson who has been trained to fit shoes and who will help you select just the right size and style for your feet. (For more shoe-buying strategies, see Chapter 8.)

Dynamic Posture Analysis—Base (Feet to Hips). Stand in front of a mirror in your normal posture without shoes. How far apart are your feet? Are they parallel, or does one foot or both feet point out at an angle? While a slight outward turn is normal, ideally your feet and knees are symmetrical and directed straight ahead. Bend your knees. Do they come over your toes, or are they more to the inside or outside of your feet?

Stand up straight. Are your knees locked? Is your weight distributed evenly between both legs? Do you fall to the inside (pronation) or outside (supination) of one or both feet? Your goal is to be equally balanced on both legs, with your knees unlocked.

Put on your walking shoes. Look at your feet, knees, and legs in the mirror. Place a small piece of masking tape or a round sticker in the center of each knee-cap and in the center of each foot, behind the toes.

Next, place your fingers on the front of your hipbones. Slide your fingers to the inside of these bones. Under your hands are the balls in the ball-and-socket joints of your hips. Point your fingers straight down toward your feet. Ideally, the pieces of tape or the stickers on your feet and knees are in straight vertical lines beneath your fingers.

Drop your arms but continue looking in the mirror. Imagine each leg, from hip to foot, as the upright of a ladder. Ideally, the rungs between your hips, knees, and ankle joints are parallel. Proceed to the next exercise.

Ladder Base into Heel-Toe Roll. Still in front of the mirror, stand with your feet as parallel as is comfortable and one shoe-width apart. This position provides maximum stability and biomechanical support for your joints. Your goal is to line up your hip, knee, and ankle joints from one side of your body to the other, creating a Ladder Base. Retraining your standing posture with your legs one shoe-width apart will help ensure a fluid stride.

From the Ladder Base, begin the Heel-Toe Roll (page 234). Swing your arms easily to add momentum to your roll and to improve your balance. Keep your knees relaxed. Pay attention to rolling down the center of your foot, just as you need to do when you're walking.

Practice rolling your feet with your knees tracking under the balls of your hips. As you roll forward, the tape on your knees should stay in line with the tape on your feet. Watch yourself in the mirror.

If you habitually lock your knees, practice this exercise for 1 to 2 minutes. Repeat it several times a day, especially when you find yourself standing in line. It will help you build dynamic strength in your knee joints so that you won't feel the need to lock them for support.

Modified Heel-Toe Roll. If your feet aren't parallel or your knees aren't tracking over your toes, you have a choice. If you're over age 60 and you're not experiencing any musculoskeletal pain in your body, you can continue walking just as you are. Otherwise, you can correct your walk by practicing the Modified Heel-Toe Roll. This exercise can be especially helpful if you've been experiencing musculoskeletal pain in your spine or lower quadrant.

As you roll from heel to toe, slowly turn your toes inward, then outward, then inward again. Make sure that your knees are tracking over your toes and your feet are parallel. Practice this for 1 minute at a time, 3 to 5 times during your walking workouts.

Gradually add more of these 1-minute intervals to your walks, provided you're not experiencing any pain. It's important not to force your legs into this new position too quickly. You could develop joint pain unnecessarily. Based on your age and flexibility level, your musculoskeletal system may need many months to realign properly. Give it the time it needs.

DBX Focus. Concentrate on your foot position whenever you're practicing the exercises in Chapter 34.

Kinesthetic Images for Week 5

Practice these frequently each day this week to experience your body in new ways.

Ladder Base. Bring this image of your hips, knees, and ankles being in alignment into your body as you stand and walk. Stand tall from your hips upward. Extend your energy from your hips downward through your legs and into the Earth.

Power Legs. Continue to be aware of the power in the legs of dancers and athletes. Bring the perception of strength into your legs, especially when you're pushing off during your walks.

Rocking Horse. While walking, picture the bottoms of your feet as being curved like the base of a rocking horse. Roll down the center of each foot from heel to toes, as described earlier.

Goals for Week 5

1. Become aware of how you use your legs while walking, standing, and sitting.
2. Slowly bring your legs into a stronger, more biomechanically efficient posture.
3. Listen carefully to your body.
4. Make changes at a speed that achieves your goals without creating stress.

WEEK 6: HARNESSING PELVIC POWER

If you notice these signs: Can't elevate your heart rate for an aerobic workout; slow pace when walking

You'll practice these exercises: Force Field/Kick Sand; Power Surge/Pelvic Push-Off; DBX Focus

You'll experience these benefits: Increasing your walking speed; building more thrust for speed bursts; feeling more grounded; improving balance; strengthening your legs; contouring your buttocks

You'll achieve this training goal: Building pelvic power

If legs are the workhorses of the body, then the pelvis is the engine that gives them power. We can only build strong legs and a strong walk by connecting with our core.

While in Japan one summer, I trained in the traditional Japanese arts of tea ceremony, calligraphy, Noh (masked dancing), *budo* (swordplay), and flower arranging. Each class began by focusing attention in the center of the body. The center, often referred to as the *hara*, is the point of consciousness from which all movement flows. It is also the center of balance. Whether I held a sword, a fan, or a calligraphy brush, connecting with my center empowered all of my actions.

Over the past 5 weeks, you've become more aware of your postural habits in your daily activities, improved your biomechanics, and sharpened your walking technique. You've learned how to avoid potential injuries and to fall in step with Mother Nature's design. Your efforts so far have been rewarded with increasing elegance, efficiency, and ease when you move.

You're now ready to begin building power and speed in your walk. In week 6, you'll learn to direct your core strength through your legs into the ground beneath and behind you. By focusing your energy, you'll build thrust, like a rocket.

Exercises for Week 6

Repeat these frequently each day this week to build new muscle memory.

Force Field/Kick Sand. Picture a circle beneath your body, with two-thirds of the area being directly under and behind your body. This circle represents the Force Field where you'll have the greatest contact with the ground and therefore the greatest thrust.

To increase your push-off power, practice standing tall on one leg. With the other leg, scrape the ground as if to kick sand beneath and behind you, like a dog digging a hole. Use your whole leg from the hip, not just your knee. Feel the action up into your buttock. Repeat six times on each side.

Apply this push-off power when walking. Walk tall. Keep yourself directly over your Force Field for maxi-

mum traction and speed.

Power Surge/Pelvic Push-Off. You'll need a partner for this exercise. Have the person place a long, wide band low across your pelvis, at your hipbones. As she holds the ends behind you, walk naturally for 30 seconds. Then she should add resistance by pulling on the band.

Keep your upper body relaxed. Don't muscle up in your arms and chest or tighten your jaw. Sink into your legs and push off from behind, as if kicking sand. Continue for another 30 to 45 seconds.

At this point, your partner should let go of one end of the band. When she does, don't slow down. Surge forward with your newly discovered push-off power. Use your ankles fully as you roll your feet forward. Walk dynamically for 30 seconds. Then repeat the exercise.

DBX Focus. Concentrate on the hip and leg stretches (DBX #6 through #13) in Chapter 34.

Kinesthetic Images for Week 6

Practice these frequently each day this week to experience your body in new ways, especially while you are walking.

Power Surge. Picture a racehorse at the starting gate. When the bell rings, the horse surges forth. Notice how its hooves throw dirt to the rear as it speeds along.

Power Legs. Continue to observe the legs of dancers, athletes, and running animals. Feel their agile power in your legs. Watch martial artists like Jackie Chan and Michelle Yeoh. They maintain their balance in their centers at all times. When they deliver a blow, energy shoots outward at lightning speed from their cores through their extremities. Their legs are powerful in action, stable at rest, like tamed tigers. Cultivate greater awareness of your own leg power.

Goals for Week 6

1. Discover how your legs can more fully support you in all positions.
2. Build leg strength as you get in and out of a chair, bed, or bathtub.
3. Use your whole body when walking. Connect the power from your pelvis to your legs.
4. Thrust the ground away from you as you walk.
5. Roll your feet forward, using a full range of motion in your ankles.

Chapter 34

THE DYNAMIC BODY EXERCISES

In the previous chapters, you learned the basic movement patterns of Dynamic Walking. You analyzed your daily activities and observed your own habits to learn how you've been growing your body. You began using gravity and other dynamic forces more consciously, as tools to rebuild your body. Now you're going to learn to apply those same forces to a more complex activity: stretching.

The 14 stretches in this chapter—I call them the Dynamic Body Exercises—have actually been a lifetime in the making. Long before I imagined that movement therapy would become my life's work, I was captivated by the grace and joy of a body in motion.

As a child, I began dancing, and I have continued ever since. I remember performing in a recital at age 5, enrolling in ballet classes shortly thereafter, winning an *American Bandstand* jitterbug contest at age 10, and attending classes in social dance as a teenager. In my lifetime, I've studied a variety of ethnic dance forms, from African to Noh, the Japanese art of masked dancing. My husband and I have even developed our own Latin fusion dance style.

For more than 25 years, I have been a student of Anna Halprin, an award-winning dancer and choreographer. When I first began my training, Halprin encouraged me to work with children, just as she had. For 7 years, I taught movement education in a Montessori school that my son was attending. I engaged my students in a variety of activities, including yoga and mime, soccer and swordplay, puppetry and masked dancing.

Maria Montessori, an Italian physician and educator, established the Montessori school system on a foundation of fun plus fundamentals. Her philosophy inspired my curriculum. For example, I taught my students roller skating, an activity that they loved (fun) and that helped them improve their posture (fundamentals). It required that they use both legs equally, glide balanced on either leg, move forward and backward, relax their upper bodies, and build lower-leg strength. My students learned to apply their roller-skating skills to other activities; they played broom hockey and choreographed dance routines on skates.

When I moved on to teaching college students and eventually to teaching adults, my experiences gave me the opportunity to watch for the universal movement patterns common to all age groups. By studying disciplines as diverse as belly dance and yoga, tai chi and cha-cha, I was able to identify a common alphabet of movements from which each person builds his body language and each culture its unique dance expression.

For example, my research taught me that the human spine is capable of five primary movements: bending forward (forward flexion), bending backward (hyperextension), bending to either side (lateral flexion), twisting to either side (rotation), and being straight (extension). The spine is healthiest when stretched in each of these positions equally and regularly, on a daily basis. All dance forms, all sports, every expression of body language derives from these five spinal positions. They're some of the most basic links among humans of all ages and ethnic backgrounds.

GETTING BACK TO BASICS

Based on what I've learned over the years, I'm convinced that this common alphabet of movements is essential to a healthy body and a peaceful soul. It is what led me to create the Dynamic Body Exercises, or DBX.

Learning the DBX is like learning your ABCs. The exercises provide the foundation not only for walking but also for more complex activities such as swinging a golf club or planting a garden. In the first few weeks of practicing the DBX, you'll learn to stretch your spine evenly in all directions; to elongate your body to feel lighter and more lifted; to breathe more fully; to stretch your five sets of leg muscles; to maximize the range of movement in your spine, shoulders, and hips; and to improve your postural alignment.

Within a couple of months, as you rebuild your posture, you'll find a "home base"—a quiet, calm center where your skeleton supports you more easily, a place of peace in gravity. You may also notice a decline in the habitual tension patterns that color your thoughts and feelings.

Many people have asked me how the DBX differ from yoga. Both exercise systems build conscious (somatic) awareness and use breathing patterns to dissolve stress, increase vitality, and generate tranquility. Personally, I prefer the DBX because they're more practical and more connected to my everyday life than yoga. I demand a lot from my stretching—a quick, commonsense routine that I can apply to my daily activities.

Through the DBX, I've learned how to avoid injuries and how to improve my strength more rapidly when weight training. The exercises have also helped me to heal my sciatic pain, improve my sports performance, and work more easily at my computer. So if anything, the DBX is a practical, everyday yoga—a mind–body technique that teaches me how to move through life with greater energy, efficiency, elegance, and ease.

The 14 stretches in the DBX are designed to complement Dynamic Walking. When used together, the two maintain the musculoskeletal system in a balanced state. The stretches change alignment; Dynamic Walking sets the new alignment.

Over time, repeating this pattern—change, set, change, set, change, set—coaxes the body into a more dynamic posture. You're poised for movement and poised at rest.

MAKING THE MOST OF YOUR WORKOUTS

When you perform the Dynamic Body Exercises, always think *FIT*—as in *Fre-quency, Intensity,* and *Time.* These three elements help determine the effectiveness of your workout and, ultimately, of the DBX.

The guidelines that follow will help you determine how often, how hard, and how long to exercise. Just remember to stay conservative, starting slowly and easily and working up gradually. Injury always sets you back. If you have a chronic condition such as diabetes, talk with your doctor before beginning this—or any—exercise program.

Frequency: For the best results, practice the DBX at least once per day for the first several months, and at least three to five times per week thereafter. You may also use the exercises as follows:

- After any stressful or unbalanced activity
- Every hour when you're seated for long periods of time
- After 5 to 10 minutes of exercise and again at the end of the workout

If it's cold or windy outside, you may want to do the DBX indoors before you begin your workout. Then repeat them once you get home.

Intensity: When you begin doing the DBX, you may notice soreness in some new places. This is an indicator that you're making the necessary structural changes for your body to realign itself. Over time, the discomfort will go away.

Keep in mind that there is a difference between soreness and pain. Exercise should never be painful in any part of your body. If any movement hurts,

immediately stop what you're doing and consult your doctor.

Time: Hold each DBX stretch for two or three breath cycles (one inhale and one exhale per cycle), or 20 to 30 seconds. Initially, the entire DBX sequence will take 12 to 15 minutes to complete. But once you become accustomed to the exercises, you'll be able to do them in 8 to 10 minutes.

Before I explain how to perform the individual DBX stretches, I want to spend some time on the ins and outs of breathing. The rhythm of your breathing should coordinate with the rhythm of the activity you're performing—in this case, the DBX. Begin and end each exercise with an awareness of your breath. Exhale fully when you're about to enter the effort phase of the movement and whenever you compress your torso. Also exhale when you want to release deeper into a stretch.

When you're inhaling, allow your torso to expand and stretch in all directions, like a balloon filling with air. Be sure to keep your shoulders down and relaxed. Use each inhalation to refocus on your form. And always inhale when returning to an upright position (spinal extension).

DBX #1: THE LONG SHIRT PULL

Everybody loves this exercise because it feels so good. And the more you do it, the faster you'll build a lighter, lifted, and younger-looking body. Adapted from ballet, the Long Shirt Pull improves postural alignment and stretches your body from head to toe. It incorporates two of the five basic spinal positions: forward flexion and extension.

THE HEEL-TOE ROLL. This movement prepares your body for the rest of the exercise. Begin by standing with your feet together. Envision your feet separated by the width of one shoe. Move your feet apart that distance, keeping them as parallel as is comfortable (A).

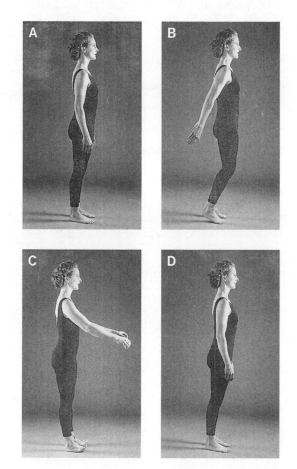

ROLL from heel to toe, rocking back and forth down the center of your feet (B, C). Imagine that your feet are curved like the base of a rocking horse. Equalize pressure on the inside and outside edges of both feet. Widen your toes as you roll onto the forefoot. Try to maintain your feet in a parallel position, but don't force them. Keep your knees gently flexed or soft. Watch in a mirror or look down to make sure that your knees are tracking over your toes. Allow your arms and shoulders to swing effortlessly.

STOP rocking and equalize the pressure on both feet (D). Move on to the Roll-Down.

THE ROLL-DOWN. Tuck your chin to your chest (E). Exhale and slowly roll down toward the ground (F). Keep your knees relaxed and aligned over your middle toes. If you have lower-back problems, rest your forearms on your thighs for support and stretch from there. Inhale, exhale, and relax while your arms and head dangle loosely (G). Inhale and exhale again, releasing all tension. Proceed to the Roll-Up.

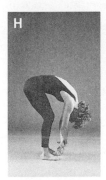
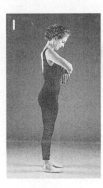
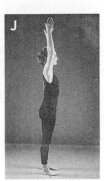

THE ROLL-UP. From the Roll-Down, very gently cross your arms at the wrists (H). Imagine that you're pulling a shirt up and off your body. Inhale as you roll up, with your arms relaxed, your elbows leading, your hands gliding along the front of your body (I). Lift the imaginary shirt up over your head, stretching upward (J). Keep your head level. Don't arch your back. Move on to the Returning to Extension.

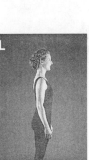
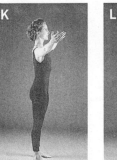

RETURNING TO EXTENSION. Grow taller through your spine as you release your arms and shoulders. Keep your pinkies in your peripheral vision (K). As you continue moving your arms down to your sides, feel your shoulders drop into a settled place, like a shirt hanging effortlessly on a hanger (L). Look around. Notice if you feel taller. Repeat twice more.

DBX #2: HYPEREXTENSION

This backward-bending stretch is one of the five spinal positions. You may already be using this position to wash your hair in the shower. Do the stretch gently, especially if you have lower-back pain. Use your breathing to relax into it.

RAISE your arms upward, lifting your torso (A). Arch your back, looking up and behind (B). Do not drop your head backward onto your shoulders. Stay lifted out of your lower back and your hips. Hold for two or three breath cycles. Return to a standing-tall position, then bring your arms and shoulders down. Let them hang relaxed at your sides (C). Move on to the Shoulder Rolls.

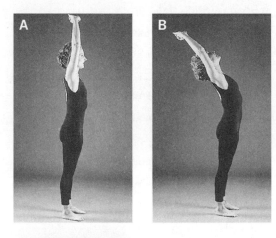

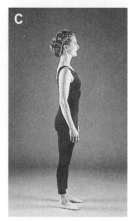

DBX #3: SHOULDER ROLLS

Have you noticed that the first six letters of *shoulder* spell the word *should*? Perhaps that's because when we "should" ourselves (as in "I should have done that"), our shoulders seem to rise up around our ears.

Many of us carry tension in the shoulder yoke, the area around and between the shoulders. We tend to round our shoulders as we go about our daily business—whether we're sitting at a computer, washing dishes, or driving a car. Doing this exercise can help you relax your shoulder yoke, release tension, and improve posture.

If you tend to carry your head forward, Shoulder Rolls are critical. Your head and neck cannot return to proper alignment until your shoulders are back and down. Although this exercise does not stretch the spine, it's included here because shoulder tension affects posture and spinal health.

When you start doing Shoulder Rolls, be gentle until you find your range. Your goal is to dissolve shoulder tension and allow your shoulders to rest relaxed on your rib cage, like a shirt on a hanger.

STAND tall, with your arms hanging at your sides (A). Roll your shoulders up (B), back (C), down (D), and around. Synchronize your breathing with your movement, exhaling and inhaling fully for two or three breath cycles. Wiggle your jaw to create a yawn, which can relax your jaw, neck, and shoulders. Move on to the Lateral Stretches.

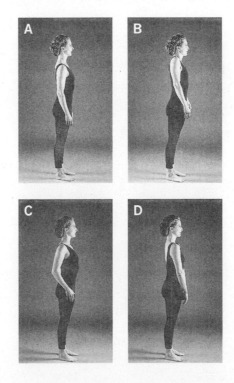

DBX #4: LATERAL STRETCHES

Many of us have a stronger arm and a dominant side to our bodies. Stretching the muscles on either side of your torso releases tension in your spine and balances your body, left to right. If you tend to carry one shoulder higher than the other, you may find that Lateral Stretches, together with Shoulder Rolls, help to level them out.

REACH overhead (A). If it's comfortable, entwine your fingers. Stretch toward the right, exhaling and lengthening both sides of your torso (B). Stay evenly balanced on both feet, pressing your left foot deep into the ground. Be careful not to twist, arch backward, or compress your spine. (Practice against a wall to find the correct position.) Extend out through your arms and the top of your head. Breathe deeply as you release into the stretch. Find those muscles deep in your abdomen that pull you back into an upright position. Be aware of restacking the building blocks of your body. Repeat, stretching to the left side (C). Repeat to both sides once or twice more. Return to a standing-tall position to begin the Spinal Rotation.

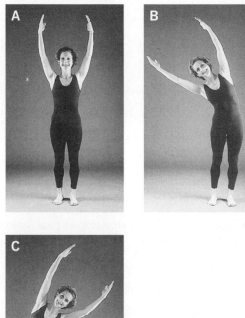

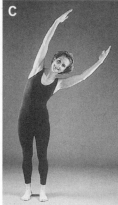

DBX #5: SPINAL ROTATION

Life doesn't always take you in a straight line. Sometimes you must navigate around corners and obstacles. This exercise makes daily activities that require you to twist your torso easier. It also makes your stride more graceful. When you walk tall, the swinging of your arms and legs naturally creates a gentle spinal rotation that massages your spine, shoulders, and hips.

When doing this exercise, notice if it's easier to rotate in one direction than the other. Balance your efforts to improve your musculoskeletal health.

STAND tall, with your feet parallel and your knees slightly bent (A). Allow your wrists and arms to float upward, to shoulder height. Raise your shoulders as you inhale, then drop them as you exhale, keeping your arms outstretched to your sides. Repeat.

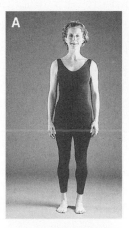
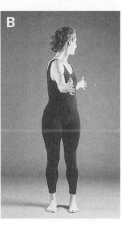

PIVOT your head from one side to the other, looking from one hand to the other. Then gently rotate your upper body, following each hand, in turn, as it moves behind you (B). Exhale as you turn, inhale as you return to center. Allow your whole upper body to enjoy the movement. Look as far behind you as possible on one side, then the other.

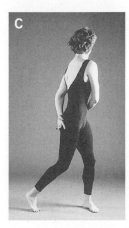

WIDEN your stance and rise up on one toe, then the other, as you rotate around (C). Relax your shoulders and let your arms drop against your sides. When you hear your arms make contact, you'll know that you have let go of the tension in your shoulders. Allowing your arms to swing free is one goal of this exercise. After 20 to 30 seconds, move directly into the Hip Stretch.

DBX #6: HIP STRETCH

Adapted from Latin dance, this exercise can help you develop independent hip action (meaning each hip moves separately from the other) and keep your pelvis young. The hip motion is vital to a natural, fluid stride. It also improves balance and prevents falls on stairs.

The Hip Stretch feels great in your lower back. If you tend to arch your back, repeat the exercise frequently during the day, especially after standing or sitting.

This stretch can be difficult for men, since their hips are often narrower and tighter than women's. If it's hard for you, prepare for it by standing with your feet together and your hands on your hips. Lift, then lower one hip at a time. You can lift your heels in turn, if necessary. Slowly widen your stance, maintaining your hip motion until you are in a slightly squatted position.

BEND at your hips and knees to drop into a squat. Place your hands on your thighs, with your fingers pointed inward (A). Keep your back straight and your shoulders down and relaxed. Lift and lower each hip by imagining that you are vigorously scratching your backside on a tree (B, C). Exhale and inhale fully in rhythm to your movements. Proceed directly into the Hamstring Stretch.

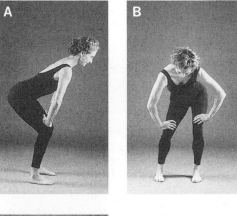

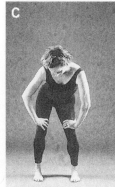

DBX #7: HAMSTRING STRETCH

This is the first of five stretches that target the leg muscles. The hamstrings are located on the back of each thigh. These muscles can be tight if you sit a lot, if your lower back is swayed, or if you stand with your knees locked or your feet wide apart. In my experience, men tend to have tighter hamstrings than women.

TURN to your right. Fold your arms and bend over to place them on your right thigh, just above your knee (A). As you exhale and relax, allow your upper-body weight to slowly straighten your right knee (B). Your right foot is pointed forward, while your left foot is at a 45-degree angle. Your left knee, whether it's bent or straight, is aligned over your left toes.

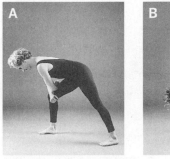
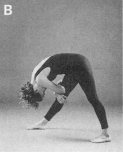
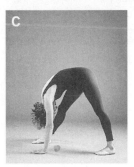

CONTINUE relaxing into this position, without pushing, through three breath cycles. As your right knee straightens, you can either drop your arms (C) or keep one hand on your shoelaces. Roll up enough to pivot to your left side to stretch your left hamstring. Be sure to keep your neck relaxed, your head dropped, and your eyes looking back behind your legs.

REPEAT the exercise to your left side. Then move directly into the Calf Stretch.

DBX #8: CALF STRETCH

Your calf muscles are located in the backs of your lower legs. They're connected to the bottoms of your feet by the Achilles tendons. Keeping your calf muscles stretched can help you avoid plantar fasciitis, a troublesome foot condition that can cause severe heel and sole pain.

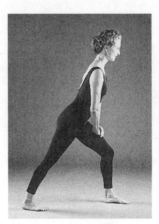

FROM the Hamstring Stretch, roll up, supporting yourself with your left hand on your left knee, if necessary. In this position, turn your right heel out so that your right foot is pointing forward, parallel to your left foot. Keep your head, neck, torso, and right leg in one long line, as if you are a plank leaning against a wall. Do not arch your back or stand upright from your waist. This puts too much pressure on your lower back. Keep your lower left leg perpendicular to the ground and your right heel pressed down. Hold this position for three breath cycles, or 20 to 30 seconds. Move on to the Soleus Stretch before repeating this stretch facing to the right.

DBX #9: SOLEUS STRETCH

Underneath the calf muscle lies the soleus muscle. It, too, can contribute to plantar fasciitis if it isn't stretched regularly and thoroughly. It tends to tighten up in women who wear high heels.

To stretch the right soleus muscle, push off on your left foot and step backward so that it's slightly in front of your right foot. Tuck your buttocks and lower yourself as if to sit, as shown. Any pressure should be behind your knees, not in your kneecaps or quadriceps (the muscles on the fronts of your thighs). Keep both knees flexed. You'll feel the broad band of your right Achilles tendon flatten out. Keep your upper body lifted, your lower back lengthened. Exhale and inhale deeply three times.

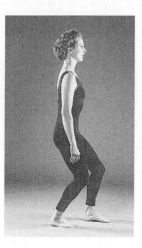

Pivot to your right. Step forward with your right foot to stretch your left calf muscle (follow the instructions for the Calf Stretch). Then push off on your right foot and move it backward so that it's slightly in front of your left foot. Repeat the Soleus Stretch, this time working your left soleus muscle. Move on to the Shin Stretch.

DBX #10: SHIN STRETCH

The shin muscles run along the outside of the shinbone, in the front of the lower leg. They are small muscles that build strength slowly when you walk (running doesn't develop them at all). They can burn when you walk briskly or when you perform the Heel-Toe Roll if you aren't used to the exercise.

This stretch works *only* when done correctly. So pay attention to proper form. This is one of the most important stretches you can do after a walking workout.

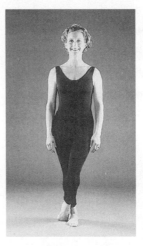

STAND tall, with your feet one shoe-width apart. Do a Heel-Toe Roll (see page 234) until you're in a balanced position, then stop.

CROSS your left foot over your right, drawing your left toes back along the outside of your right foot. Turn your left foot under so that your toes are pointing behind you, as shown. Bend your knees so that your right knee presses into your left calf. Breathe deeply, holding this position for three breath cycles, or 20 to 30 seconds. You may feel the stretch in your left shin, ankle, toes, or arch—they're all connected. Repeat on the other side.

DBX #11: QUADRICEPS STRETCH

The quadriceps muscles, located at the fronts of your thighs, can get tight from excessive sitting and poor walking technique. As the longest muscles in your body, they work with your hamstrings to help you maintain balance.

If you have poor balance, use a tree or a low fence for support when you do this stretch. You can also improve your balance by keeping your feet from falling to the inside (pronation) or the outside (supination) while walking. Wearing shoes with good support can help.

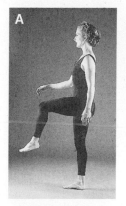
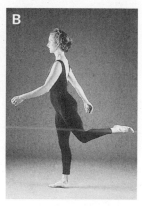
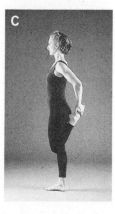

STAND on your right leg and swing your left leg like a pendulum (A, B). Drive the movement from your hip, not from your knee. Notice how you can swing your leg without scuffing the ground. That's because you're standing tall on your right leg.

REACH back and grab your left foot, or your pants leg, behind you. Pull it toward your left buttock (C). Keep your knees relaxed and your pelvis tucked under. Breathe deeply for 20 to 30 seconds. Move immediately into the Ankle Stretch. You'll stretch your right quadriceps a bit later.

Note: If you have knee problems, you can work your quadriceps in another way. Position yourself next to a sturdy, stable chair, with your right hand on the chair back for support. Standing on your right leg, begin swinging your left leg. Extend it far enough behind you that when you plant your left toes and bend your right leg, you feel a stretch in your left quadriceps muscle. Continue for 20 to 30 seconds.

DBX #12: ANKLE STRETCH

All of the weight of your upper body lands on your ankles. These joints are critical for balance and for keeping your stride vigorous and youthful.

By rolling your foot from heel to toe with each step, you keep your ankles limber and your lower legs in good condition. If you stop rolling and start walking flat-footed, you may look and feel years older.

FROM the Quadriceps Stretch, release your left leg and let it swing forward. Catch and tuck your knee to your chest (A). Lengthen your lower back and keep your torso erect. Drop your arm while keeping your left leg in place. Slowly circle your ankle in all directions (B). Move immediately to the Psoas Stretch.

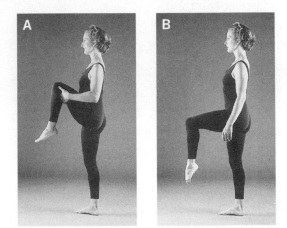

DBX #13: PSOAS STRETCH

The psoas muscle is one of the most important postural muscles and one of the longest in your body. It extends from the top of the inside of your thigh all the way up to your diaphragm, which separates your abdomen from your chest.

You began working your psoas muscle with the Quadriceps Stretch. This stretch lengthens the muscle and trains it to hold your pelvis in a neutral position. This builds core strength and lower-back support.

To get the full benefit from this exercise, follow the instructions carefully. When you lower your leg to the ground, make sure that you grow taller through your spine.

FROM the Ankle Stretch, lower your left leg to the ground (A). Continue to grow taller through your spine. Press your belly button toward your backbone, as if you are pressing your lower back against a wall (B).

Now go back and repeat the Quadriceps Stretch, Ankle Stretch, and Psoas Stretch for your right leg.

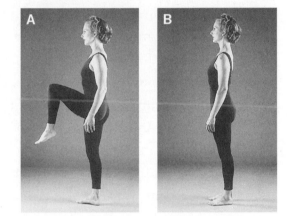

DBX #14: THE LONG SHIRT PULL

Finish the DBX series with three Long Shirt Pulls (see page 234) to balance the building blocks of your body. Notice how you feel compared with when you did your first Long Shirt Pull.

CHAPTER 35

YOUR DYNAMIC WALKING ROUTINE

Walking is a deeply nurturing activity. Its simplicity allows it to fulfill many purposes. It can provide time alone, time with a buddy, time to commune with nature, time to solve problems, time to explore new terrain, time to exercise, time to be with your kids, time to be with your dog, time to get errands done, time to travel to your next destination.

No matter why you're walking, you'll enjoy it more once you learn to do it dynamically. You'll be more deeply in tune with your body, so you'll avoid injury and get maximum benefit from every workout.

In this chapter, you'll build on what you've already learned about Dynamic Walking, applying all the fundamentals of good form to your daily walks. You'll learn awareness exercises that not only help you monitor your progress but also keep you safe during your workouts. You'll warm up and cool down safely by progressing through a variety of gears, just like an engine. And by using an efficient arm swing and other new techniques, you'll ultimately transform your walk into a fluid glide.

For each gear, I've included an approximate time frame so you'll have some idea of how long you'll need to perform the various exercises and techniques. Eventually, you'll discover your optimum time in each gear. For some walks, you may opt to stay in first gear. For others, you may hold steady in second or fourth, depending on how fast you want to travel and how many calories you want to burn.

FIRST GEAR: WARMING UP

Begin walking at a slow pace, with your arms long and swinging freely at your sides. This gives your shoulders an opportunity to unburden their load and relax. Stay lifted out of your hips to allow your legs to swing like pendulums.

Your arms will start swinging naturally, in cadence with each step. Don't force them to move. Don't carry anything in your hands. Wear a fanny pack to hold your keys, I.D., water, and the like.

While in first gear, you'll do a series of scans: the Body Scan, the Environment Scan, and the Technique Scan. You can remember them with this simple mnemonic: Together, they'll make you feel *bet*ter (as in *B*ody, *E*nvironment, and *T*echnique).

The Body Scan

This exercise gets you out of your head and into your body—fast.

Part A: Scan each part of your body, from your feet to your head. Pay attention to what you're feeling. If you notice any areas of discomfort or pain, rate each area on a scale from 1 to 10, with 1 being the most comfortable and 10 being the least. Remember this number for comparison at the end of your walk.

When you fail to acknowledge your aches and pains, you may subconsciously compensate for them, which can get you into trouble. But by paying attention to any discomfort, you can consciously experiment with the exercises you are learning to make yourself feel better.

Part B: Evaluate your vitality level, rating it on a scale from 1 (least vitalized) to 10 (most invigorated). Remember this number for comparison at the end of your walk. Depending on your goals, the outside temperature, and other factors, walking can either invigorate you or drain you. Noting how you feel, either mentally or in a logbook, can help you sort out cause and effect.

The Environment Scan

This exercise takes you outside yourself and connects you with the sights, sounds, and smells of nature.

Part A (the Eye Scan): Using only your eyes, continuously scan the path in front of you from far to near, the way you might study the road while driving. Make scanning a habit. Memorize the path. This allows you to spot obstacles and oncoming traffic well before you meet up with them. You'll feel safer because you're less likely to trip and fall. Your body will relax, your head will remain lifted and level, and you'll walk tall. Looking down strains your neck, shoulder, and back muscles and restricts breathing.

Part B: Once you've memorized the path, you are free to scan the rest of your surroundings—to enjoy the beauty of nature, to soak up the vitality of the air, and to appreciate being alive and having the gift of walking the Earth. Repeat the Eye Scan frequently. It's an important practice, especially when you're increasing your speed, hiking on uneven terrain, or walking on a crowded street.

The Technique Scan

This exercise brings you back to your body and sets your intention for your training walk.

Part A: Do several Short Shirt Pulls (page 208) as you walk. Bring the lift into your torso. Stretch tall out of your hips. Become aware of the weight of your arms and legs. Let them swing like pendulums from your shoulders and hips. Use their momentum to power your walk. Use your ankles through their full range of motion. Imagine the

bottom of each foot curved like a rocking horse. Roll along the length of your foot, from heel to toe. As you roll onto your forefoot, be sure to relax and spread your toes. Clenching them could cause bunions.

Balance your right and left sides, distributing your weight equally between your right and left legs. If you have new shoes, they should help stop you from collapsing your feet toward the insteps (pronating) or to the outside (supinating). Balance your arm swing, too. A dominant arm swing or leg push is a repetitive stress that could eventually twist your spine.

Practicing the Heel-Toe Roll (page 234) has made you more aware of the position of your knees over your toes. By making sure your knees track correctly, you diminish wear and tear on these joints, so they're good for more mileage over the course of a lifetime.

Part B: If you followed the 6-week program outlined in Chapter 33, you've already done several analyses of your posture and stride. Mentally review what you discovered about your body. For example, you may have realized that your upper body was positioned behind your lower body. If so, you practiced the

Rib Cage Slide (page 221). Do that now as you walk. Notice your results.

Every week, choose only one or two corrections on which to focus while you walk. Write your results in a walking log. By concentrating on only one or two things per week, you'll feel less overwhelmed and better able to track the changes that are occurring throughout your body.

DBX STRETCH BREAK

If you're like most people, your body needs 8 to 10 minutes to warm up. So once you've warmed up in first gear, stop and stretch using the Dynamic Body Exercises in Chapter 34. Stretching now will help dissolve the habitual tension patterns that you've brought with you on the trail. It will also bring your body back into balance. You'll probably notice a dramatic increase in the speed, ease, and efficiency of your walk. (If it's cold or windy outside, stretch gently at home before beginning your workout.)

After stretching, resume walking in first gear. Quickly repeat the three scans to observe any changes and to refocus your intentions.

SECOND GEAR: PICKING UP THE PACE

In first gear, your arms were swinging at your sides. In second gear, they'll be bent at the elbows and pumping. But if you move them into position before your legs are fully warmed up, two things could happen: You may never release your shoulder tension, and you may not get maximum effort from your legs. It's your legs' job, not your arms', to power your walk.

In second gear, you want to increase the power of your push-off. First, you need to find your optimum stride length. To do this, practice walking with a too long stride (overstriding) for 30 seconds. Notice how you bounce and how that feels in your joints and lower back. Now switch to tiny steps for 30 seconds. Feel the tension in your hips and notice the lack of a pendulum swing in your legs.

Next, lengthen your stride slightly, still keeping your feet in the Force Field (page 228) beneath and behind you. Take shorter, quicker steps with a rapid turnover. Practice the Kick Sand exercise (page 228). Remember the feeling of the Pelvic Push-Off (page 228) and use that to power your walk.

Once you've maxed out the power of your legs, your arms will naturally bend at the elbows to create a shorter, more efficient pendulum. The arm stroke itself is very clean and precise. Your arms swing naturally from your shoulders, with each one bent at about a 90-degree angle and moving in a fist-to-hip, elbow-to-hip pattern. Don't cross your arms over the center line of your body or pump them up and down to burn extra calories. This creates shoulder tension and is counterproductive.

To propel yourself forward, put power into the backward phase of the arm stroke. Imagine flames shooting from each elbow equally. Relax and recover on the forward phase of the swing.

Stay in second gear for 2 to 5 minutes before moving on to third gear.

THIRD GEAR: PRIMING YOUR HIPS

You'll spend only 20 to 30 seconds of your walk in third gear. It warms up your hips in preparation for fourth gear, when you really pick up your pace.

Begin with a walking Short Shirt Pull (page 208) to increase the lift out of your hips. Then slow your pace to keep from tripping. Visualize a line down the center of the path you're on. Cross each foot *over* the line to make your hips swivel. (This is a training technique used by racewalkers.) You can clasp your fingers together at waist height to help maintain your coordination.

FOURTH GEAR: HITTING TOP SPEED

As you move into fourth gear, stop crossing your feet over that imaginary center line, but keep the image of the line in your mind. The inside edge of each foot will just touch the center line.

As you approach your top speed, the momentum of your legs will naturally swivel your hips. People who carry more weight around their hips swivel more easily than those who are thin. Nevertheless, if you stay lifted out of your hips, your legs and feet will naturally fall into a more proper alignment along that center line. In fact, one of my clients, who had difficulty flexing her ankle and lifting her toes because of an injury, was able to avoid chronically stubbing her toes by swiveling her hips, which brought her foot into proper position.

While you're in fourth gear, quickly repeat the Body Scan, Environment Scan, and Technique Scan. Occasionally take short, quick steps to increase your steps per minute and to become more aerobic. Resist taking longer strides. A bouncy walk could cause heel and knee pain.

If your shins start burning, stop to do the Shin Stretch (page 244). Then proceed at a slightly slower pace and build slowly in intervals. Interval training involves alternating periods of brisk walking with periods of recovery. In this case, walk fast for 1 to 2 minutes, then slow down for 1 to 2 minutes. Repeat this pattern 3 to 5 times. By gradually increasing the exertion phase and decreasing the recovery phase, you can safely build power and speed. Slow down if you begin to lose form.

Within a few months, you'll be able to stay in fourth gear for at least 20 minutes, all the while maintaining speed and proper form. Once you have mastered the Dynamic Walking technique (or your weight has stabilized if weight loss is your goal), you may prefer to do most of your maintenance walking in second gear.

WINDING DOWN FROM YOUR WALK

Once you've finished your walk, downshift into first gear and cool down for 5 minutes. Do a final Body Scan, paying special attention to any areas of your body that were painful or tense when you first started out. Notice any change in how you feel. Reassess your vitality level, too.

Reserve the last segment of your workout for repeating the DBX exercises. Eventually, you'll be able to do the entire series in just 8 to 10 minutes, as each muscle group learns to relax and stretch quickly. If you forgot to do your final scans while you were cooling down, now is a good time to fit them in.

TUNING IN TO YOUR INNER COACH

Now that I've showed you the principles and techniques of Dynamic Walking, I want you to continue your training with another coach, the most important coach you'll ever have, the one living inside you. That coach is available to you 24 hours a day at no charge, and knows your habits intimately. Ask for your inner coach's advice whenever you need it.

Especially when you're starting your training, your ego may step in and want to do things another way. It can fill your head with thoughts like "I don't really need to work out today" or "It's not really hot; I can leave my water bottle at home" or "I've got to fit into those jeans, so I'll push myself just a little harder." Eventually, your inner coach will be empowered enough to challenge these thoughts and make decisions that are in the interest of your whole body. A patient, positive, nonjudgmental attitude works best when building skills to last a lifetime.

CHANGING PAIN TO PLEASURE

Just as your inner coach can help you learn and hone your Dynamic Walking technique, your coach can also teach you to listen to your body "speaking" to you through sensations of pain and pleasure. These are normal, healthy messages—a sort of biofeedback.

One of the goals of Dynamic Walking is to decrease pain and increase pleasure for a lifetime through correct alignment and biomechanics. As you progress, don't be alarmed if you experience discomfort in new places. As your musculoskeletal system rebalances, as your body transforms, pains may shift around.

Experiment with the exercises I've given you and observe the results. Reread the instructions often to make sure that you're performing the movements properly. Over time, your efforts will be rewarded with greater pleasure—and a happier body.

Something else will happen that's just as magical: As you continue walking dynamically, your stride will transform into a glide—elegant, efficient, and easy. When the glide takes over, you feel as though you can go on forever. Your body may feel more fluid and integrated, too. You'll move in a smooth, relaxed manner at any speed, in any situation, even when entering a room full of people. You'll feel more confident, more in control. And that will have a positive impact on all areas of your life.

Happy trails. Walk with beauty.

—*Dr. Suki Munsell*

To learn more about Dynamic Walking, or to request information about other fitness programs and training, visit the Dynamic Health and Fitness Institute's Web site at www.dynamicwalking.com or call 888-852-6717.

Part VIII

EVERYTHING ELSE
YOU NEED TO KNOW

CHAPTER 36

COMMON QUESTIONS
ABOUT WALKING

Many walking questions come up over and over again. They're the ones featured in this chapter. As you read through them, perhaps you'll find information that you can apply to a situation or problem that you're experiencing.

BACK TO BASICS

Q: What's the best time of day to walk?

A: It varies from one person to the next. In the summer, some people love to walk in the mornings, when it's nice and cool and the sun is up early. In the winter, it may be a good idea to walk on your lunch hour, since that's the warmest part of the day. The fresh air revitalizes you for the afternoon, plus you get a healthy dose of vitamin D from the sun's rays. Your diabetes will likely enter into this decision, as walking will affect your blood sugar. Test before and after exercise, and talk with your doctor about it. The question is, when are you most willing and able to walk? That's the best time for you.

Q: Should I eat before I walk and during my walk?

A: Again, it varies from one person to the next. "It's important to check your blood sugar level before and after you exercise because people respond differently to exercise," says Kashif Munir, MD, an endocrinologist and medical director of the Joslin Diabetes Center at Baltimore Washington Medical Center in Glen Burnie, Maryland. "Some people's blood sugar levels will drop during exercise, so a small snack such as an apple or a sports drink with 15 to 20 grams of carbohydrate will provide needed carbohydrates and keep your blood sugar level from dropping too low. For other people, their blood sugar levels might actually transiently rise, so they wouldn't want to eat anything or even drink a sports drink.

"If you're exercising for more than an hour, you should check your blood sugar level every hour, maybe even every half hour," Dr. Munir adds. "Keep a carbohydrate snack, such as some juice, on hand to correct low blood sugar."

Also be sure to drink a nice, tall glass of water before you head out, especially first thing in the morning. Your body may be somewhat dehydrated after a night's sleep. Dehydration is especially dangerous for people with diabetes because it can increase blood sugar levels.

Q: *What's the simplest way to determine how fast I'm walking?*

A: The easiest way to gauge your speed without wearing a pedometer—or getting in your car and measuring mileage, which can be pretty difficult unless you walk along a street—is to count your number of steps per minute. The experts use this number to calculate pace, based on an average stride length of 2$\frac{1}{2}$ feet. (Stride length is the distance from the heel of one foot to the heel of the other foot when you're taking a step.) They've already done the math for you.

- 70 steps per minute equals 30 minutes per mile, or 2 miles per hour.
- 105 steps per minute equals 20 minutes per mile, or 3 miles per hour.
- 140 steps per minute equals 15 minutes per mile, or 4 miles per hour.

If you pay attention to your steps, after a while, you'll be able to estimate your pace fairly accurately without bothering to count. You'll just know what a 20-minute mile or a 15-minute mile feels like.

Q: *How many calories do I burn by walking a mile?*

A: The average 150-pound person burns between 80 and 100 calories per mile. That number can change depending on your height, your weight, your fitness level, whether you're walking on hills or level terrain, what you're wearing, the outside temperature, and many other factors.

If your goal is to lose weight, forget about the numbers. Instead, develop a healthy eating plan that you can live with, and incorporate as much physical activity into your daily routine as possible. Walk for at least a half hour a day. If you can do more, great! Maybe you can squeeze in a half hour in the morning and another half hour in the evening. Then during the day, take as many short walks as you can, indoors or out.

Become aware of how much time you spend sitting, and make an effort to fill some of those minutes with physical activity. At work, for example, pace around while you're talking on the phone and use the restroom on another floor or in the farthest corner of your building. That way, you know you're burning more calories throughout the day. The exact number doesn't really matter.

SHOE SAVVY

Q: *My walking shoes have two sets of eyelets. Which should I use?*

A: That extra set of eyelets allows you to fine-tune the fit of your walking shoe. If you have a narrow heel, lace both sets of eyelets to tighten the top of your shoe. This keeps your heel from slipping, so you don't develop blisters. You may have to experiment to get the lacing just right.

Q: *I walk early in the morning, so my walking shoes always get wet. They're still damp the next day when I go to put them on. Any suggestions?*

A: Buy a second pair of walking shoes, so you can alternate between them. People with diabetes should never walk in wet shoes. "First of all there is the risk for blistering or ulceration due to friction," says Robert Katz, DPM, a podiatrist in Bradenton, Florida. "And secondly there is an increased risk for developing some type of infection such as athlete's foot."

While you're wearing your second pair of shoes, stuff newspaper inside your wet shoes to help soak up moisture, so they might dry faster. Just don't put wet leather shoes near a heat source. Drying them too fast causes them to shrink or crack.

Q: When should I get new shoes?

A: Replace your walking shoes every 6 months or 600 miles, whichever comes first. At that point, it doesn't matter if the shoes still look great. They've lost a lot of their cushioning power. Be kind to your feet, and you'll keep walking forever.

FOCUS ON FITNESS

Q: How can I evaluate my fitness level as a walker?

A: James Rippe, MD, a cardiologist, founder and director of the Rippe Lifestyle Institute, and author of *Dr. James Rippe's Complete Book of Fitness Walking*, has developed a special formula to help walkers assess their fitness. Find a flat 1-mile loop. Warm up for 5 minutes, stretching your calves and hamstrings. Then walk the mile as quickly as you can without running out of steam. Compare your time against the benchmark for your age group.

- Under 30: If you can walk a mile in 13 minutes, you're in great shape.

- 30 to 39: Doing a 14-minute mile puts you in the "great shape" category.

- 40 to 49: Cover a mile in just under 15 minutes (14 minutes, 42 seconds), and you're at the top level of fitness for your age group.

- 50 to 69: Doing a 15-minute mile is excellent.

- 70 or over: If you can walk a mile in 18 minutes, 18 seconds, you're very fit for your age.

If you exceed the ideal time for your age group by 3 to 6 minutes, you're not in the best shape aerobically. But don't worry—just keep walking. Regular, consistent exercise can lower your time.

Q: Is it possible to do too much walking? Can I overtrain?

A: If you're new to walking, build up your time and mileage gradually. After all, you want your body to get used to the exertion. You may not actually hurt yourself, but if you feel stiff and sore, it may keep you from going out again.

If you're walking regularly and you're really picking up your pace, you can just as easily overtrain. Here are some indicators that you may need to reduce your intensity or distance or even take a day off once in a while.

- Your daily walks seem to be getting harder instead of easier.
- You feel more tired than usual during the day.
- You have difficulty springing out of bed in the morning.
- You have trouble falling asleep or sleeping soundly.
- You begin eating less or eating irregularly.

If you cut back on your walking routine and your symptoms persist, see your doctor. There may be an underlying medical problem that's making you feel bad.

STAYING INJURY FREE

Q: My hands swell when I walk. Is this a problem? It feels funny, and I don't like it.

A: Swelling in your hands is normal. When you swing your arms, the blood rushes down into your fingers. It isn't harmful, but it could be uncomfortable, especially if you wear rings. It's a good idea to take off your rings before you go walking.

If the swelling bothers you, try squeezing your hands into fists from time to time while you walk. This helps push blood back from the fingers. Some people carry small rubber balls to squeeze. Keeping your elbows bent as you swing your arms can also minimize swelling. But unless you're racewalking, the bent-elbow technique can feel rather silly.

Q: Whenever I start walking, I get side stitches. What causes them, and what can I do about them?

A: A side stitch—a sudden, stabbing pain in your side—results from a spasm of the diaphragm, the muscle that separates your chest and abdomen. It's crying out for oxygen because your expanded lungs and contracted abdomen are blocking normal bloodflow. This sounds serious, but it's not a big deal.

At the first sign of a side stitch, stop walking. Using three fingers, massage the area where the pain is most severe until you feel relief. Do not hold your breath. As your breathing slows to its normal rate, the pain should subside. Then you can resume your walk. Like any muscle, your diaphragm cramps when it isn't warmed up properly. So remember to warm up before you head out. Walking slowly should do the trick.

Q: Help! I'm having pain in the fronts of my lower legs. What is it?

A: It sounds like shin splints, a common problem among beginning walkers. It results from doing too much too soon. Your shin and calf muscles cramp from overuse, and you notice a burning pain in your shins.

To avoid shin splints, increase your distance and pace gradually, and always take time to warm up before doing any speedwork. If you've already overdone it, try slowing your pace. If you're still in pain, try stretching your calf muscles. Stand facing the nearest wall or tree, then lean forward, putting your palms against the wall or tree and keeping your heels flat on the ground. Or sit on a bench with your legs straight out in front of you and flex your feet toward you.

Still in pain? Hobble home and apply ice for 15 minutes. Be sure to wrap the ice in a towel, to protect your skin from the cold.

Q: I have heel pain. What should I do?

A: Heel pain becomes increasingly common with age, especially among the over-40 crowd. Often it results from a condition called *plantar fasciitis*—that's inflammation of the plantar fascia, a sheath of connective tissue that runs along the bottom of the foot. As this tissue becomes overstretched and inflamed, it produces sharp pain, especially first thing in the morning when you get out of bed. The pain eases as you walk around, but it can come back, especially if you sit for a long time.

As you get older, your body's tissues become less pliable. That's why stretching is so important. For heel pain, stretching your calf muscles may help. If it doesn't, you may need better walking shoes or special shoe inserts (called *orthotics*) to keep your ankles from rolling inward (overpronating), which may overstretch and inflame the plantar fascia.

However, since any foot pain can be serious for someone with diabetes, schedule an appointment with a podiatrist. You need to find out what's causing your pain. If you keep stretching and tearing your plantar fascia, you may develop heel spurs, painful bony protuberances from the heel bones.

Q: *How can I avoid blisters?*

A: Blisters spell big-time trouble for people with diabetes. Here's how to keep your feet blister free.

- Wear clean socks. Choose high-tech socks made from fibers that wick away moisture. Skip the cotton and look for synthetic blends such as Coolmax or Wonderspun.

- Make sure that your shoes fit both of your feet. Often one foot is larger than the other. The friction created by wearing the wrong-size shoe—whether it's too small or too large—can lead to blisters.

- Check your shoes regularly for things that could injure your feet, such as frayed material, tacks poking through, and pebbles.

- Use powder such as Zeasorb on your feet to help them stay dry. "Keep your feet as dry as possible if you have diabetes," says John M. Giurini, DPM, president-elect of the American College of Foot and Ankle Surgeons and associate professor in surgery at Harvard Medical School in Boston. "If your feet are wet, you're more likely to get blisters, because there's more friction, and any time you have an open sore on your foot it can lead to a bacterial infection."

- "If you have diabetes and you get a blister, you need to be a detective and figure out why you got it," says Dr. Giurini. "A blister on the side or top of the foot is usually shoe related. Is the shoe too tight, loose, narrow, or rigid? A blister on the bottom of the foot is usually because there's too much sliding within the shoe. Is the shoe too loose or not laced tightly enough?"

- "If you get a blister, get out of that shoe and off that foot, treat the blister with an antiseptic medication such as Neosporin, and put a sterile dressing over it," says Dr. Giurini. "Watch the blister for 1 to 2 days. If it's not getting better, or if it's getting worse and you see redness or discharge or smell a foul odor, see a doctor immediately."

SAFETY FIRST

Q: *There are some nasty-looking dogs in my neighborhood, and they're not always chained or fenced in. What can I do to protect myself?*

A: You're right to be concerned. Even dogs that seem friendly around their owners can become aggressive when they're protecting their turf from strangers. If you can take another route, do so. Or call local authorities— either your town's animal-control officer or the police—to find out the provisions of municipal leash laws and to report any violations.

If you must walk by a property with potentially dangerous dogs, be sure to carry something for protection. Tie a sweatshirt around your waist, wear a fanny pack, carry an umbrella or a walking stick—anything that you can put between yourself and a dog, in case one tries to bite you. The dog won't care if he gets you or the object in your hand. As he bites down on the object, keep tension on it and back yourself to a place of safety, like inside a car or behind a fence. Then let go and wait for him to leave.

Never stare down a dog. Instead, stand still and try to stay calm. Say, "No!" in a deep, firm voice. If the dog stops in his tracks, yell, "Go home!"

If a dog knocks you down, curl into a tight ball and protect your head and neck with your hands. Wait for the animal to leave, then slowly move to safety. Running will only attract the dog's attention.

Report any attack to your local animal-control office immediately. Even if the dog bit your fanny pack and didn't harm you, he's dangerous, and his owner should be notified.

Q: *I like walking on an outdoor track near where I live because I don't have to contend with dogs or cars, but I get bored. Any suggestions?*

A: An outdoor track can be lots of fun for walking. It's a great place to interval train—speed up for one lap, slow down for the next. You can listen to music during your workouts since you're out of harm's way. (If you're completely alone, you might want to keep one ear free, so you can hear a stranger approaching.) You can practice special techniques, such as walking with your feet parallel to one of the white lane lines or crossing each foot over the line to stretch out your hips.

Wear a watch or a stopwatch to monitor your pace. If you walked a 15-minute mile last week, can you shave a few seconds off your time this week? Write down your times, so you can track your progress.

When you're on a track, you can really let your mind wander since you shouldn't have to watch for obstacles. Carry a little tape recorder to record your brainstorms or to make tapes to send to relatives or friends. If you're comfortable walking with someone, just having a buddy can distract you from the monotony of going around in circles.

PAIRING UP TO WORK OUT

Q: *My wife and I like to walk together, but she has trouble keeping up with my brisk pace. I don't want to give up our time with each other, but I do want to get a workout. What should I do?*

A: Your situation is quite common among walking couples. Each person has a different pace or a different stride, so one gets bored slowing down or the other suffers trying to keep up. There isn't any perfect solution, but since you're the faster partner, you could wear a weighted vest or backpack while you're walking. Or you could try using a PowerBelt. It's a device that you wear around your waist, with handles to pull for an upper-body workout. Just pumping your arms helps to rev up your heart. (For more information on the PowerBelt, see Chapter 19.)

Perhaps the best suggestion is for you to do most of your workout first, then join your partner for your cooldown. You'll be relaxed and in a great mood by the time you're finished walking, ready to share quality time with your partner.

Q: *I want to start a walking club in my area. Where do I begin?*

A: Do you really want to add this kind of complication to your life? Getting an entire group together on a regular basis is very difficult.

On the other hand, you may find some interest in walking classes. Many people are willing to pay a nominal fee to have someone motivate them to walk. If you're willing to lead a class, all you need is a watch, a cell phone, CPR certification, and some enthusiasm. You don't have to know racewalking technique, although good posture is definitely a plus.

To find your recruits, place an ad in your local newspaper or post a notice at your church or YMCA. Explain that you'll lead walks at a particular time, from a designated starting point, a set number of times a week for a fee of $3 to $5 per session. (If you're experienced in racewalking technique or you have some sort of training certification, you may want to charge more.) You'll have the walking group you wanted in the first place, and as a bonus, you'll be getting paid for your efforts.

The catch is, you're responsible for everything, including getting your walkers back to the starting point on time, making sure that they stay within their target heart-rate ranges, and leading them in stretches before and after every workout. You may want to have water bottles or light snacks available, too.

As you can see, this approach takes work. But it may be more plausible and inviting than trying to recruit members for a walking group.

TREADMILL TIPS

Q: Do I get as good a workout when I'm on my treadmill as when I go outdoors?

A: All treadmills are different. Some give very accurate indications of your speed, while others don't. What's more, when you're on a treadmill, the walking surface is continuously pulling away from you. As a result, you're not getting the solid push-off from your back foot that you do when you're walking outside.

But the real issue is that you're probably using the treadmill for a certain reason—perhaps you don't feel safe walking outside, or the weather is keeping you inside. What's important is that you're moving your muscles, burning calories, and getting a great workout.

You might not want to do all of your walking on a treadmill. The benefits of walking outside in nature are just too great to ignore. So make sure that you exercise outdoors whenever you can.

Q: *I feel dizzy when I get off my treadmill. Is there something wrong with me?*

A: Absolutely not. When you're walking on a treadmill, your body gets confused because it's moving but the scenery isn't changing. So once you return to terra firma, your body thinks it should keep going, even though you're standing still. To minimize dizziness, try slowing your treadmill to a very easy pace before you hop off. Then walk around for a few minutes until your sense of equilibrium returns.

Photo Credits

© Hilmar: pages 113 to 118, 120 to 121, and 148 to 151

© Mitch Mandel/Rodale Images: pages 153 to 163

© John Ruth Sterling: pages 36 to 37

© Jeanette Vonier/Elegant Images: pages 234 to 247

Index

Boldface page references indicate photographs. Underscored references indicate boxed text.